Adolescent Pregnancy and Parenting

Jean-Victor P. Wittenberg
Daniel F. Becker • Lois T. Flaherty
Editors

Adolescent Pregnancy and Parenting

Reducing Stigma and Improving Outcomes

Springer

Editors
Jean-Victor P. Wittenberg
University of Toronto
The Hospital for Sick Children
Toronto, ON, Canada

Daniel F. Becker
University of California San Francisco
San Francisco, CA, USA

Lois T. Flaherty
Cambridge Health Alliance
Harvard University
Cambridge, MA, USA

GAP Committee on Adolescence

ISBN 978-3-031-42501-1 ISBN 978-3-031-42502-8 (eBook)
https://doi.org/10.1007/978-3-031-42502-8

This Springer imprint is published by the registered company Springer Nature Switzerland AG
The registered company address is: Gewerbestrasse 11, 6330 Cham, Switzerland

Paper in this product is recyclable.

Preface

In 1986, members of the GAP Committee on Adolescence published the monograph *Crisis in Adolescence, Teenage Pregnancy: Impact on Adolescent Development*. This monograph extends the previous work of the committee. It reviews findings from a number of fields to update our understanding of influences, interventions, and outcomes for both teen parents and their babies. While the earlier monograph focused on negative outcomes and viewed pregnancy and motherhood as factors derailing healthy adolescent development and placing babies at risk, reflecting the predominant views at that time, this one examines social and familial factors that support or interfere with optimal development of teens who become pregnant and those who become parents in the light of new research and new understanding of the role of social context both as a risk factor and a determinant of outcome. Each chapter addresses specific, albeit overlapping, perspectives and fields of knowledge. In particular we focus on the influence of stigma as a predictor of undesirable outcomes for both parents and babies.

Although authors are individually responsible for their own chapters, all participants in the Committee met twice annually face-to-face and several times annually by teleconference. Thus we had the opportunity and the luxury of discussing each other's work as we wove this monograph together. Authors came from the US and from Canada, from the ranks of trainees and veterans, both female and male. Areas of particular interest ranged from focuses on adolescents to infants, from systems to individual experience, from psychological development to social policy. We have tried to overcome our own subtle sources of bias and the stigma that emanates from it to present a comprehensive and up-to-date review of the field. Individual authors reached their own conclusions in their own papers and participated in our overall conclusions documented in the final paper.

Throughout our work, we have been fortunate to have a consultant for our committee who has contributed in a major way to our work by articulating her own lived experience of being a teen mother and experiencing the stigma attached to this situation. She has guided and accompanied our exploration and helped us to learn our own biases. Her perspectives are present implicitly in the thinking and concepts that structure the papers themselves.

Our intention is to help physicians and other healthcare providers, social services providers, educators, religious leaders, and policy makers reflect on the values and attitudes that influence the services they deliver, the goals they seek, and the outcomes for this particularly vulnerable sector of our communities. We also hope to empower the teens and their families to help them change the power differential that maintains stigma.

Toronto, ON, Canada — Jean-Victor P. Wittenberg
San Francisco, CA, USA — Daniel F. Becker
Cambridge, MA, USA — Lois T. Flaherty

Introduction

Adolescent pregnancy and the babies of teen mothers have been a focus for social attention and concern for many reasons and for many years. The overwhelming emphasis has been on prevention, and although many prevention initiatives, such as increased access to reproductive health care, have been very successful, there has been relatively little effort directed toward supporting and enhancing the mothering capability of those young women who elect to keep their babies. This book will focus primarily on how we as a society, and as clinicians, tend to help or hurt teen moms by our attitudes and behaviors that decrease or increase stigma.

Teen sexuality, pregnancy, and parenthood often excite moralistic disapproval, although the degree, manifestations, and consequences of that disapproval vary across many different parameters. For example, there are different attitudes to teen pregnancy in different regions of the US [9]. There are different attitudes depending on family and ethnic background. Like other behaviors that are often the focus of social disapproval, there are associated health risks for the newborn as well as to the mother and father. We ask if it may be that in at least some of those cases disapproving, demeaning, and rejecting day-to-day interpersonal interactions are in themselves pathogenic. That is, the stress they impose—that of stigma—causes toxic stress to young parents and to their babies.

The introduction to the 1986 monograph stated its overarching concern:

> Pregnancy at any age engenders developmental change; in the immature it creates developmental crisis. Pregnancy during adolescence thus compounds the stresses of two normative developmental stages and endangers the successful resolution of either one. … Among crises during adolescence, pregnancy endangers not only the individual and society, but also the unborn child [4, p. xix].

It has been over 30 years since those lines were penned. A great deal of new knowledge has been generated. Social attitudes have changed and yet there is evidence that social attitudes continue to discredit and unfairly discriminate against pregnant teens and their babies—along with many other groups and individuals. For example, highly respected organizations that pride themselves on taking a moral stance and sincerely oppose discrimination implicitly demean pregnant teens and, as a result, their babies. For example we can see in the following statements that the

Centers for Disease Control and the American Academy of Child and Adolescent Psychiatry both implicitly communicate that teen pregnancy is a pathological condition.

> In 2010, teen pregnancy and childbirth accounted for at least $9.4 billion in costs to U.S. taxpayers for increased health care and foster care, increased incarceration rates among children of teen parents, and lost tax revenue because of lower educational attainment and income among teen mothers [3].

> If pregnancy occurs, teenagers and their families deserve honest and sensitive counseling about options available to them, from abortion to adoption. Special support systems, including consultation with a child and adolescent psychiatrist when needed, should be available to help the teenager throughout the pregnancy, the birth, and the decision about whether to keep the infant or give it up for adoption. There may be times when the pregnant teenager's emotional reactions and mental state will require referral to a qualified mental health professional [2].

Pressures within our communities continue to advocate approaches and policies that are likely to discriminate against this very vulnerable group [6]. The time seems at hand to re-examine our attitudes and their impact.

Pregnant teens and their offspring remain of concern, but as is so often the case, more knowledge has made our understanding of the situation more complex. Although some teen mothers seem to do well, the outcomes for many are less desirable. Many show evidence of negative short, medium, and long-term health and mental health outcomes [8]. The data on infant development confirm concerns; the infants tend not to do as well than those born to older mothers. They have lower birth weights, a significantly higher infant mortality rate, and are more likely to end up as adolescent mothers themselves (ibid.). These babies also show challenges to optimal development and school readiness.

There is a strong belief in professional, political, and public sectors that having a baby in adolescence blights the lives of teen-aged girls. Some studies, however, like those that examine the longer-term trajectory of young women's lives, suggest that for many women having a baby in adolescence was not a roadblock to development and in fact may have spurred a more adaptive and constructive posture and outcome compared to their socio-economic peers. This ironic finding—that some adolescent girls find better life trajectories as a result of pregnancy but have babies who are disadvantaged—may also be understood at least in part, as a result of negative social attitudes, i.e., stigma. Are our social attitudes directly hurting babies and young mothers? We are convinced that stigma is a significant predictor of adverse outcomes for many teens and their babies and that many would do better were it not for the impact of social disapprobation.

The chapter on the *Voices of Lived Experience* includes narratives of young mothers, fathers, and their children. We hear firsthand accounts of parental experiences before, during, and after the pregnancies. Stigma is a universal experience although different individuals handle the stresses of their situations more or less adaptively. Their voices echo throughout the chapters that follow as well. This chapter includes two detailed first-person accounts, one of a teen mother and another of a teen father, each of which illustrates the extraordinary capacity of two young parents to cope with adversity. While each is a tale of resiliency, each also illustrates the challenges faced by young parents in completing their education, confronting negative stereotypes, dealing with low expectations, and overcoming barriers to accessing services. There are also several shorter vignettes to illustrate specific issues for teen mothers and babies as well as one from the child of a teen parent.

In the third chapter, we present a discussion of stigma as it has been researched and formulated in fields of sociology, psychology, and economics. We describe how stigma imposes stress on those who are its object, how that stress predicates adverse health outcomes, and how pervasively it is expressed and experienced in daily interactions in families, public circumstances, activities of daily living, healthcare services, education, research, and policy. We review research on the influence of stress on development, decision-making, and parenting for adolescents who are at developmentally vulnerable periods in their lives. We explore the impact of stigma as it affects disadvantaged children and teens before pregnancy, during pregnancy, and afterwards as they become parents. We explore the impact of stressed young parents on the unborn fetus and on the baby and child in their care. Stigma impacts fetal, infant, child, and adolescent development in the realms of cognition, emotional regulation, social relationships, vocational achievement, physical and mental health, etc. Finally we turn to an examination of how social policy influences stigma; how policy keeps stigma in place and protects the powerful or changes it to permit greater compassion for all members of our communities.

Power differentials are central to the influence of stigma. Negative misattributions can of course be held by any individuals or groups toward others. They have lasting and negative impacts, however, when they are exercised by the individual or group that has power. Stigma is effective because of the power of group beliefs against a weaker subgroup [5]. The beliefs are held to provide some advantages to the group in power. When power relationships are changed, outcomes are changed. For example higher rates of depression in women vs. men are reduced when women have more power within a society [7]. It has been argued that the 1964 Civil Rights Act by prohibiting segregation in healthcare facilities decreased the power differential and increased access to services, thus leading to substantially reduced numbers of infant deaths in the Black population [1]. The consequences are costly to us all. To reduce or eradicate the adverse effects of stigma the power differentials must be addressed. The nature of the issues and problems associated with stigma and its impact on teen parents and their babies is explored in the subsequent chapters.

The fourth chapter addresses development in adolescence, with particular emphasis on the impact of stress. In this chapter we review the psychology and neurobiology of adolescent development, the capacity of teens to manage stress, and the imposition of stress secondary to stigma on teens and their functioning as parents. We understand that adolescence is a period of change which may or may not be tumultuous. It is the phase of life in which we establish an identity, a sense of self that guides us through the years of adulthood, the years in which we are given adult responsibilities and authority, including the responsibility and authority to bear and raise children. In some ways our physical capacities outrace our psychological capacities. We can take sometimes life-threatening risks before we learn to consider their consequences. We can bear children before we may be ready to raise them. In this chapter we focus on the development of the ability to effectively solve problems (*executive function*) for oneself and for another (an infant) in the context of our teen psychological development. How well can the teen parent maintain the ability to problem solve (EF)—and a sense of another's mind, *reflective function* (RF)—particularly under the weight of social pressures, such as peer pressure and social stigma? We review the relevant knowledge about adolescent brain development.

The fifth chapter is devoted to young fathers. An understudied group, they are nonetheless vital in the lives of young mothers and their babies. We look at the factors involved in early fatherhood, the various relationships these young men have with the mothers of their children and their children, and ways in which these relationships can be optimized to support children.

In the sixth chapter, we address infant development, and we examine psychological and neurobiological development in infancy and the early years, infants' needs for parenting relationships, and the impact of stress in infancy whether it be transmitted by parental stresses or directly to the infants themselves from other stress-inducing experiences. This chapter considers the outcomes for infants of teen mothers. The knowledge in the field of infant development has grown exponentially over the past quarter century. The critical importance of experiences in the early years of life in determining life outcomes is reviewed. In addition, the authors examine the interface between social and psychological experiences and their biological impact. In this field we find early answers that address the toxic consequences of excessive stress and we begin to elucidate the conflict between our desired goals for all members of our communities, including teen parents and their babies, and the measurable impact of our social attitudes. We also begin a discussion on the development and influence of RF—the capacity to envision mental states in self and others. We accord a high degree of significance to RF in that it mediates healthy parenting, it grows out of social interactions, it provides an internal system for personal regulation, and it fails under stress. We think about the impact of stigma, a stress-inducing social pressure that may lead individuals to default to non-RF thinking and interacting.

The seventh chapter focuses on interventions to support pregnant and parenting teens and their babies and the evidence that validates them. We consider the ways in which social beliefs affect conceptualizations of what is helpful and interventions designed to prevent pregnancy or subsequent pregnancy in teens.

Chapters 8 and 9 provide an overview of psychiatric disorders and treatment. The peripartum period is a time of risk for psychiatric disorders in women of all ages, and many adolescents who become pregnant either have pre-existing disorders or develop them perinatally. Treatment of the pregnant adolescent is complex and involves careful evaluation of risks and benefits, as well as attention to the adolescent's social and cultural context.

Chapter 10 considers implications of the previous chapters for public policy.

Finally we offer conclusions and recommendations that are directed to mental health service providers, the healthcare, education, and social service communities, and to policy makers and legislators. We encourage all of these groups to consider the impact of their own beliefs and the possibility that stigma is embedded in their own service delivery patterns.

University of Toronto
Toronto, ON, Canada
Hospital for Sick Children
Toronto, ON, Canada

Jean-Victor P. Wittenberg

References

1. Almond DV, Chay KY, Greenstone M. Civil rights, the war on poverty, and Black-White convergence in infant mortality in the rural South and Mississippi. December 31, 2006. MIT economics working paper 07–04. Retrieved from: https://ssrn.com/abstract=961021
2. American Academy of Child and Adolescent Psychiatry. Facts for families. When children have children. Washington, DC: Author; 2012. Retrieved from https://www.aacap.org/App_Themes/AACAP/docs/facts_for_families/31_when_children_have_children.pdf
3. Centers for Disease Control. About teen pregnancy. Atlanta: Author; 2017. Retrieved from https://www.cdc.gov/teenpregnancy/about/index.htm
4. Group for the Advancement of Psychiatry, Committee on Adolescence. Crises of adolescence. Teenage pregnancy: impact on adolescent development. New York: Brunner/Mazel; 1986.
5. Hatzenbuehler ML, Phelan JC, Link BG. Stigma as a fundamental cause of population health inequalities. A J Public Health. 2013;103(5):813–21.
6. Porter E. Politicians push marriage, but that's not what would help children. New York Times, March 23, 2016. Retrieved from https://www.nytimes.com/2016/03/23/business/for-the-sake-of-the-children-not-marriage-but-help.html
7. Seedat S, Scott KM, Angermeyer MC, Berglund P, Bromet EJ, Brugha TS, et al. Cross-national associations between gender and mental disorders in the World Mental Health Organization World Mental Health Surveys. Arch Gen Psychiatry. 2009;66(7):785–95.
8. Swann C, Bowe K, McCormick G, Kosmin M. Teenage pregnancy and parenthood: a review of reviews 2003. Evidence briefing. London: Health Development Agency; 2003.
9. Talbot M. Red sex, blue sex: evangelical teens and pregnancy. The New Yorker, November 3, 2008. Retrieved from https://www.newyorker.com/magazine/2008/11/03/red-sex-blue-sex

Contents

Epidemiology, Trends, and Public Policy

1

Daniel F. Becker

Teen birth rates vary widely around the globe and over time. Globally, the teen birth rate has fallen by about half since 1960, from 86 to 43 per 1000. Although accurate data are not available from all countries, the data we do have indicate teen birth rates are generally much higher in developing nations than in developed countries.[1] Within the developing world, rates are highest in Sub-Saharan Africa, averaging 100 per 1000 (with rates as high as nearly 200 per 1000 in some nations), and lowest in Southeast Asia and the Pacific (approximately 23 per 1000). Most births to women 15–19 years old in the developing world involve women in marriages or committed relationships; child marriage is still prevalent in many countries, and exists in the USA as well. In general, teen birth rates are higher in rural areas, in poorer countries, and in areas riven by conflict [20]. Rates in developing nations tend to be higher among less educated women [16]. Complications of pregnancy and childbirth are the leading cause of death and disability among women of reproductive age in developing countries [16].

More extensive data exist with respect to the developed parts of the world. Here, again, considerable rate variability is evident geographically—with the USA having the highest teen birth rate at 37.9 per 1000, Canada having less than half that rate, and the Netherlands having the lowest rate, at 4.1 per 1000 [20].

---

[1] Adolescent fertility rates are based on data on registered live births from vital registration systems or, in the absence of such systems, from censuses or sample surveys. The estimated rates are generally considered reliable measures of fertility in the recent past. Where no empirical information on age-specific fertility rates is available, a model is used to estimate the share of births to adolescents. For countries without vital registration systems fertility rates are generally based on extrapolations from trends observed in censuses or surveys from earlier years [20].

D. F. Becker (✉)
University of California San Francisco, San Francisco, CA, USA
e-mail: Daniel.Becker@ucsf.edu

J.-V. P. Wittenberg et al. (eds.), *Adolescent Pregnancy and Parenting*,
https://doi.org/10.1007/978-3-031-42502-8_1

Birth rates have been recorded reliably in the USA since the middle of the last century. Data for teen birth rates by race/ethnicity in the USA have been available beginning in about 1990. USA rates declined very slightly during the 1970s and the early 1980s—then increased during the late 1980s, peaking in the early 1990s (at about 60 per 1000). Furstenburg [7] has pointed out that teen pregnancy rates have always been high in the USA, but this needs to take into account marriage statistics. Starting in the 1960s, fewer pregnant teens entered marriages. This trend began among Black teens, and later spread to white teenagers and older women, who came to see that "single parenthood was at least as viable a solution to premarital pregnancy as was a hasty marriage or its alternatives (informal adoption or illegal abortion)" [7, p. 11]. Therefore, what really changed were marriage rates, and these have changed for women of all ages, not only teenagers.

After the peak in the 1990s, US teen birth rates began a steady overall decline [6, 8]. The teen birth rate went down by 50% between 1990 and 2010. In 1991, the USA teen birth rate was 61.8 births for every 1000 adolescent females, compared with 26.5 births for every 1000 adolescent females in 2013, and 17 in 2019.

Non-Hispanic white, non-Hispanic Black, and Hispanic groups have all shown generally declining rates—with the non-Hispanic Black rate showing the most substantial decrease during this period. Nonetheless, rates among both non-Hispanic Black and Hispanic teens are still substantially higher than those among whites [11]. Recently, the highest teen birth rate has been among the Hispanic group, at 28.9 per 1000 in 2017 [11]—although this is well below the 1991 rate of 104.6 per 1000 [9]. Still, as noted above, the USA teen birth rate is higher than that of many other developed countries, including Canada and the United Kingdom [10].

Wide geographic variation is observed within the USA—with Arkansas having the highest rate, at 32.8 per 1000, and New Hampshire having the lowest, at 8.9 per 1000 in 2017 [3].

Sociocultural Influences

There is considerable evidence supporting the importance of sociocultural influences on teen birth rates [21]. Rates are higher among those young women who are socially and economically disadvantaged—and among those whose male partners are older than they are [6]. States where conservative religious beliefs are prevalent have the highest teen pregnancy rates, even after controlling for income levels and rates of abortion [17]. Researchers have hypothesized that teens from conservative religious backgrounds who have sexual intercourse tend not to use contraceptives and not to resort to abortion if they become pregnant. The potentially complex relationships between religious adherence, political orientation, sexual attitudes, and sexual behaviors were explored in the popular press in an article titled "Red Sex, Blue Sex"—within the context of a high-profile teenage pregnancy—near the close of the 2008 USA presidential campaign [18]. The author drew on sociological research to describe stark differences in attitudes towards premarital sex, sex education, and unwed pregnancy between social conservatives and liberals. Socially conservative individuals were likely to promote abstinence-only education and condemn premarital sex, but at the same time, were supportive of pregnancy and the decision to have a baby. Liberals (and teenagers growing up in a liberal environment) were more likely to endorse delaying sex, using contraception, and having an abortion if the adolescent became pregnant. Most strikingly, the stigma attached to the pregnancy was greater among people living in "blue states" or states that tend to vote Democratic. The differences were in part attributed to the higher aspirations of teenagers in Democratically leaning states, such that educational plans were more likely to be derailed by an unplanned pregnancy.

The Role of Social Disadvantage

A considerable body of research reveals that social disadvantage predicts higher rates of teen births. This has generated the hypothesis that teen motherhood is related to the diminished opportunities available to socially disadvantaged teens. Motherhood is seen as an achievable goal that confers some social advantages, or "part of an alternative life-course strategy created in response to socioenvironmental constraints" [2]. Unlike their more advantaged counterparts, disadvantaged young women may not perceive early childbearing as an obstacle to a bright future; indeed, they may perceive it as one of a few viable paths to adulthood.

The importance of social disadvantage is of particular concern at the present time when we see social gradients between rich and poor at peak levels and rising. Social gradients refer to disparities in health outcomes between populations that differ in terms of socioeconomic status—those who are more disadvantaged have worse health (and shorter lives) than those who are more advantaged. We know that high social gradients are associated with poor outcomes and significantly higher economic and social costs for the entire community. Social capital, a construct encompassing cooperation among families, neighborhoods, and communities, has also been found to be linked to teen pregnancy rates, with higher levels of social capital associated with lower teen pregnancy rates [5]. A review of the literature on social determinants, published from 1995 through 2011, found support for other community level factors; neighborhoods with various kinds of disadvantage, including underemployment, low income, low educational levels, physical disorder, and income inequality had the highest rates of teen pregnancy [12].

The Role of Contraception and Abortion in Reducing Teen Births

While the availability of contraception and abortion has played a role in the declining birth rate among adolescents, reduced sexual activity has also been important. One study found reduced sexual activity and increased contraceptive use explain 35% and 65%, respectively, of the recent decline in teen childbearing [8]. This study also noted that policies aimed at making welfare less attractive, changing the availability of abortion and low-cost contraception did not adequately explain geographic variability in teen birth rates—suggesting, in addition, the importance of cultural dimensions. For example, non-marital teen births are more frequent among women of low socioeconomic status when they live in areas having greater levels of educational and economic inequality, suggesting that social marginalization and hopelessness may be a crucial factor [8]. Thus, policies aimed at more abstinence education and increased accessibility of contraception potentially ignore the underlying causes of teen behavioral changes.

There has been considerable research devoted to studying differences between Black and white teenagers with respect to their attitudes towards pregnancy and child-rearing. Furstenberg [7] has noted that Black teenagers and young women led the trend towards not marrying, but that they were followed by white women. The highest rates for pregnancy in both groups are in the late teens and early 20s. Black women also have rates of abortion that are twice as high as whites. Based on their study comparing over 900 Black and white teenagers, Barber and colleagues found that Blacks tended to have earlier sexual debuts and less effective use of contraception [1]. Black teens were less likely to insist that partners use condoms or refuse sex if they thought it would make their partner angry. Religiosity and poverty were important factors for both groups. Many of the women had negative attitudes towards non-marital sex and childbearing, but nonetheless had positive expectations once they became pregnant. The authors speculated that decreased opportunity costs—the reduced likelihood that having a child would interfere with life chances—were an important factor for both groups, but especially for Black teens. Many Black teens had negative attitudes towards contraception, which these and other authors have attributed to the legacy of enforced sterilization, and which was still in effect in the latter part of the twentieth century [19].

The Role of Public Policy

During Clinton's presidency in the 1990s, conservative and moderate legislators joined forces to implement welfare reform, in the belief that overly generous benefits were creating dependency and among other things, contributing to rising teen birth rates. In actuality, teen birth rates were declining, but teen pregnancy was considered a root cause of poverty, and it was widely believed that welfare provided incentives for teenagers to have children outside of marriage. The Personal Responsibility and Work Opportunity Reconciliation Act of 1996 (PRWORA), passed by Congress and signed by President Clinton in 1996, was touted as a way to "end welfare as we know it." It required states to reduce benefits by making them time-limited and contingent on seeking employment or participating in job training programs. Unmarried mothers were particularly targeted, with PRWORA including measures to encourage marriage between parents, require mothers to identify the fathers of their children, and require fathers to provide child support. The title of the act with its emphasis upon "Personal Responsibility" may have connoted the view that it is individual failure and irresponsibility that leads to poverty. As part of PRWORA, the federal program previously known as Aid to Families with Dependent Children (AFDC) was replaced by Temporary Assistance to Needy Families (TANF). TANF required states to try to establish paternity of children born to unmarried mothers, as well as to enforce collections of child support payments through a variety of measures. For example, the State Department could deny or revoke passports to individuals owing more than $5000 in child support. PRWORA requires states to submit written documentation of their goals and strategies to reduce non-marital pregnancies and births, even offering a financial incentive of $20 million each to five states with the largest declines in their "illegitimacy ratios" and abortion rates [15]. This incentive has resulted in states making abortions more inaccessible and legally punishing childbearing by not granting more assistance to families even after the number of children increases [15].

TANF allocated funds to states in the form of block grants, allowing the states flexibility in spending the money if they complied with the requirements of the Act. If they did not spend all the money in the block grant on payments to needy families, they could use it in other ways (college scholarships, for example). PRWORA had the effect of greatly reducing the number of welfare recipients while expanding the number of people living in poverty. The number of children living in extreme poverty, defined as a household income below 50% of the poverty line, increased, with a sharper increase among Black families [13]. There has not been any evidence that these austere policies have influenced teen pregnancy rates.

Birth rates among some populations may have been influenced by restrictive laws regarding abortion and contraception [21]. An example of how increased access to contraception—rather than reduced financial support is linked to lower birth rates can be seen in reviewing state policies which correlate to the sociocultural characteristics of a state's population. A study of birth rates in various states from 2000 to 2006 showed that states that implemented Medicaid family planning waivers had much larger declines in teen birth rates than those that implemented abstinence-only programs [14, 21]. For example, when comparing California and Texas, two states with comparable demographic characteristics and similar teen birth rates in 2000, birth rates declined by 46% in California compared to only 19% in Texas. Both states have large Black and Hispanic populations, but California implemented increased access to contraception while Texas relied on abstinence programs.

A review of state policies in effect in the USA in 2008 found that sex education was required in only 35 of 50 states; furthermore, 28 states required the teaching of abstinence as the only method of pregnancy prevention, while only 18 states required teaching about contraception. In 33 states, teaching about contraception is either not mandated or there is no policy (though, this does not mean that it is not taught: Massachusetts, for example, leaves this up to individual school districts). Is there a correlation between state policy on the teaching of contraception and access to abortion and teen birth rates? Interestingly, there did not seem to be one, although higher birth rates did correlate with restrictive abortion policies, suggesting again that other factors–social and cultural—played a larger role [4]. It seems likely that sex education alone would not be enough to make a difference, and furthermore the quality of the sex education that was provided is not known. What is generally termed comprehensive sex education or evidence-based sex education, which we will discuss later, is probably a necessary if not sufficient condition for pregnancy prevention.

There has been a trend away from sexuality education in schools across the USA [15]: "The percentage of schools requiring instruction about human sexuality fell from 67% in 2000 to 48% in 2014, while the share requiring instruction about HIV prevention declined from 64% to 41%. By 2014, 50% of middle schools and junior high schools and 76% of high schools taught abstinence as the best way to avoid pregnancy, HIV, and STDs. Only 23% of junior high schools and 61% of high schools taught methods of birth control generally, while 10% of middle school and junior high school teachers and 35% of high school teachers taught specifically about the correct use of condoms." These researchers conclude that in countries where adolescents routinely have access to comprehensive sex education and other social supports, teen pregnancy and birth rates are much lower than they are in the USA

The Role of Stigma

Much of the impetus behind some of these public policy initiatives can be understood in the context of stigma against teens who become pregnant: blaming them for making bad choices, and, especially in the case of Black teens, accusing them of deliberately becoming pregnant to gain welfare benefits. However, a view that is more reflective of reality may be that teenagers who bear children are embedded in a social and cultural context that limits their sense of agency. This view will be explored in the subsequent chapters. Sociocultural factors such as neighborhoods characterized by underemployment, poverty, low income, low educational levels, physical disorder, and income inequality are sources of stress for young people. For those who bring children into the world, stigma increases their stress load, makes their lives more difficult, and their parenting more challenging. The next chapter describes the voices of young mothers, fathers, and their children. We hear first-hand accounts of parental experiences before, during, and after the pregnancies. Stigma is a universal experience although different individuals handle the stresses of their situations more or less adaptively. Their voices echo throughout the chapters that follow as well.

References

1. Barber JS, Yarger JE, Gatny HH. Black-White differences in attitudes related to pregnancy among young women. Demography. 2015;52(3):751–86. https://doi.org/10.1007/s13524-015-0391-4.
2. Burton L. Teenage childbearing as an alternative life-course strategy in multigeneration black families. Hum Nat. 1990;1(2):123–43.
3. Centers for Disease Control and Prevention. Teen birth rate by state, 2017. Atlanta: Author; 2017. https://www.cdc.gov/nchs/pressroom/sosmap/teen-births/teenbirths.htm.
4. Chevrette M, Abenhaim HA. Do state-based policies have an impact on teen birth rates and teen abortion rates in the United States? J Pediatr Adolesc Gynecol. 2015;28(5):354–61. https://doi.org/10.1016/j.jpag.2014.10.006.
5. Crosby R, Holtgrave DR. The protective value of social capital against teen pregnancy: a state-level analysis. J Adolesc Health. 2006;38:556–9.
6. Darroch JE. Adolescent pregnancy trends and demographics. Curr Women's Health Rep. 2001;1:102–10.
7. Furstenberg FF. Destinies of the disadvantaged: the politics of teen childbearing. New York: Russell Sage Foundation; 2010.
8. Kearney MS, Levine PB. Why is the teen birth rate in the United States so high and why does it matter? J Econ Perspect. 2012;26:141–66.
9. Kost K, Henshaw S, Carlin L. U.S. teenage pregnancies, births and abortions: national and State trends and trends by race and ethnicity. New York: Guttmacher Institute; 2010, Retrieved from http://www.guttmacher.org/pubs/USTPtrends.pdf
10. Office of Adolescent Health, Department of Health and Human Services; 2016.
11. Office of Adolescent Health. Trends in teen pregnancy and childbearing; 2019. Retrieved from https://www.hhs.gov/ash/oah/adolescent-development/reproductive-health-and-teen-pregnancy/teen-pregnancy-and-childbearing/trends/index.html
12. Penman-Aguilar A, Carter M, Snead MC, Kourtis AP. Socioeconomic disadvantage as a social determinant of teen childbearing in the U.S. Public Health Rep. 2013;128(Suppl 1):5–22.
13. Pimpare S. Welfare reform at 15 and the state of policy analysis. Soc Work. 2013;58(1):53–62.
14. Santelli J, Kirby D. State policy effects on teen fertility and evidence-based policies. J Adolesc Health. 2010;46(6):515–6. https://doi.org/10.1016/j.jadohealth.2010.03.023.
15. Santelli JS, Kantor LM, Grilo SA, Speizer IS, Lindberg LD, Heitel J, et al. Abstinence-only-until-marriage: an updated review of U.S. policies and programs and their impact. J Adolesc Health. 2017;61(3):273–80. https://doi.org/10.1016/j.jadohealth.2017.05.031.
16. Singh S. Adolescent childbearing in developing countries: a global review. Stud Fam Plan. 1998;29:117–36.
17. Strayhorn JM, Strayhorn JC. Religiosity and teen birth rate in the United States. Reprod Health. 2009;17:6–14.
18. Talbot M. Red sex, blue sex: why do so many evangelical teen-agers become pregnant? The New Yorker, November 3, 2008. http://www.newyorker.com/reporting/2008/11/03/081103fa_fact_talbot. Accessed 12 Oct 2012.
19. Threadcraft S. Intimate justice: the Black female body and the body politic. New York: Oxford University Press; 2016.
20. United Nations Population Division, World Population Prospects. Adolescent fertility rate (births per 1,000 women ages 15–19). Retrieved from United Nations Population Division, World Population Prospects; 2019. website: https://data.worldbank.org/indicator/SP.ADO.TFRT
21. Yang Z, Gaydos LM. Reasons for and challenges of recent increases in teen birth rates: a study of family planning service policies and demographic changes at the state level. J Adolesc Health. 2010;46(6):517–24. https://doi.org/10.1016/j.jadohealth.2010.03.021.

Voices of Lived Experience

2

Natasha Vianna and Lois T. Flaherty

Introduction

While much has been written about teen parents, we seldom hear from these parents and their children themselves. The three women whose stories follow generously shared their experiences with us throughout our deliberations and contributed first-person accounts.

In previous chapters we reviewed the epidemiology of teen pregnancy and showed how it disproportionately effects poor and minority women. We described how their problems are linked to disadvantaged social circumstances and adverse experiences, and are compounded by stigma. In this chapter, we hear from teen moms and the child of a teen mom in their own words about their struggles and ultimate successes.

Teen Success, Inc., a nonprofit organization that supports teen parents, notes three common misconceptions about young mothers: (1) They can't perform well in school, (2) they have ruined their lives forever, and (3) they can't be good parents.[1]

The following stories challenge these misconceptions.

Natasha's Story: Living Between Two Worlds

If someone told me when I was 16 that I would soon become a teenage mother, I would have rolled my eyes and thought that would never happen to me. I'd heard what people said about teen moms and why they got pregnant. I also knew that I

[1] https://www.teensuccess.org/blog/3-common-misconceptions-about-teen-parents

N. Vianna
NoTeenShame.org, Oakland, CA, USA

L. T. Flaherty (✉)
Harvard Medical School and Cambridge Health Alliance, Cambridge, MA, USA

J.-V. P. Wittenberg et al. (eds.), *Adolescent Pregnancy and Parenting*,
https://doi.org/10.1007/978-3-031-42502-8_2

wasn't any of those things and I didn't make those kinds of mistakes. Fast forward to a year later when I find myself sitting on the phone with a nurse who repeated over and over into the phone "you're pregnant."

It was my junior year of high school and I went to the doctor that day for symptoms of what turned out to be a urinary tract infection. They prescribed me some antibiotics and walked me to the door. At the very last moment, the doctor asked, just to be sure, if there was any chance I could be pregnant. Confidently, I said no. She said she would do a urine test just to be sure but that I was okay to leave.

On the bus ride home, I got a call from the nurse who asked me if I was alone. I wasn't, but I knew that nobody would ask that kind of question to share good news. They had tested my urine and a pregnancy test came back positive. My heart sank and I asked over and over if it was possible this could be true. I can't remember much of what I thought at that point. Most of my body was consumed with a paralyzing fear of what this meant for myself, my future, what my parents would say, what people would think, and how my boyfriend would react.

There was also a small part of me that felt a new sense of importance. I instantly had a new responsibility or something to think about separate from my current reality.

Most people didn't know that I had been struggling with depression for about 5 years. The first time my mother took me to a doctor about my depression at maybe 12 or 13. I was crying every single night in bed and struggling to get any sleep. In the doctor's office, the only symptoms I could articulate were constantly feeling sad and hopeless. My mother decided that maybe taking some time to be away from my current reality would help, so she took me to Brazil for two months to be closer to family, in warmer weather, where I'd have a lot of new things to do and see.

The brief moments of joy I experienced in Brazil ceased when I returned back to the USA. I spiraled right back into depression. I didn't have the language to describe it then, but I'd seen and experienced domestic violence as a child. For years, I did everything I could to stay strong and pretend those things didn't affect me. For my mother's sake, I wouldn't ask or talk about it. This was possibly in fear of how she'd respond or maybe because I just didn't want to remember. I never made it into therapy—seeking mental health support was too stigmatized at the time.

For those 5 years, I was on a frequent rollercoaster of emotions. At times feeling hopeless and invisible, wondering if anyone would care or notice if I was gone. Before I was 16, I had already twice tried to end my life. I was 16 when I was sexually assaulted by a man more than twice my age. He was a friend of the family whom I was supposed to trust. I felt a part of me die that day. I felt a part of my relationship with my body and my family end. I grew angry wondering why his forced apology was validated, but my pain silenced. That wasn't the first traumatic thing to happen to me, but it was a point in my life when I was trying to fix my relationship with my body and self. It was a moment when I felt like I lost control.

Looking back, it's not a surprise that I got pregnant soon after. I was not as careful as I could have been. I also realize that there was so much about sex and reproduction that I didn't truly understand, owing to not having received adequate information. But the truth is that there was a large part of me that stopped caring what would happen to me too. Both the experiences of violation and the feeling of hopelessness made me feel that life would be better if it weren't in my own control. I put my future into the hands of whoever was willing to plan it for me.

The news of my pregnancy hit my parents hard. Both were immigrants who moved to Boston in the early 80s and quickly jumped into lives of working multiple jobs to provide for their three kids. As the only people in their families to leave their country to "make it" in the USA, they shared lots of stories with me of the sacrifices they made and expectations they had for their kids in America. My memories include watching them thrive as multi-lingual people, but also hearing their English framed as "bad English" by other people, who pressured them to shorten their names.

Ten years after immigrating to the USA, my parents divorced. I was seven. From that moment on, I did what I could to help and take some of the burden of raising us off my mother's shoulder. I took on responsibilities around the house by 11, started working to help pay for some of my expenses by 14, and made sure that I was an honor roll student in high school throughout it all. On paper, everything I was accomplishing was exactly what parents would hope for their daughter. But there was still so much turmoil inside of me.

When I found out I was pregnant and told my mother, she couldn't find words. She sat silently staring back. I left that room not having heard a word back from my mother. Just complete silence. I went back to my room wondering if that was better than hearing a lecture or words of anger. But what I truly wished for was some guidance or something along the lines of, "Okay. Let's talk about this. What happened? What do we need to do?" In all of the movies I have ever watched, an "I'm pregnant" statement was always met with either extreme happiness or extreme shock. In this situation, I got nothing. And I didn't know how to feel about it.

Hoping for a different reaction than my mom, I told my school nurse that I was pregnant. I'd spent a lot of time in her office prior to this, mostly for horrible PMS days. Unfortunately, she didn't have any wise words for me, no words of support either. And by the next day, my whole school knew I was pregnant. The nurse told my teachers, who told other teachers, who gossiped about it in front of students, who told other students. I knew everyone knew because no one made eye contact, but looked straight at my belly. Some of my teachers nodded their heads or made indirect comments about mistakes and irresponsibility.

I considered having an abortion. I was in a Catholic high school, the nurse knew that I was thinking about abortion, and I wondered if she had told people about my pregnancy so I wouldn't get one. Now that everyone knew I was pregnant, they'd know what I did if my belly didn't start to grow. I worried that people would talk about me as they did about other girls who got abortions. They were called sluts. Eventually, the nun in my school pulled me aside to remind me that "abortion is wrong" and that my soul could not be saved from that kind of mistake. That week in theology class, my teacher even assigned my class an essay topic: abortion. We were to write about it and read it to the class.

Before my belly began to grow, I had once again experienced a moment where choice and autonomy over my body were being pulled away from me. I felt tugging from my school and peers to make decisions they felt were better for me.

Looking back at those first few weeks of pregnancy, my life at 17 wasn't much different than my prior years not pregnant as a teen. I had been looking for the power I needed to make the best choice for myself and my own body, but that choice kept being taken from me. Before the end of my first trimester, more decisions were made for me: my parents canceled my prenatal appointments, angrily kicked me out, telling me to live with my boyfriend, and stopped paying my high school tuition. In a matter of 2 weeks, not only did I have to think about preparing for this pregnancy, I had to find ways to get healthcare again, move in with somebody I didn't want to spend my life with, and find a way to finish my education.

Moving in with my daughter's father was a challenge. We found out I was pregnant just a few weeks before he left for the Marine Corps. From my 9th week to the week I would give birth, he wouldn't see my belly, attend any appointments, or be present for the entire experience. I would, essentially, do this whole thing by myself.

I was working a part-time job after school and on the weekends. I took a few weeks off after I found out I was pregnant to work on issues. When I returned, my boss said, "I'm glad you took care of that problem and you're back." I had to awkwardly explain that the "problem" he was referring to was still growing inside me. Embarrassed at making an assumption, but still curious enough to continue snooping into my life, he simply asked what my plan was now. The plan was to pick up more hours and work full time over the summer since I needed the money to feed myself and had nothing else to do with that time.

Finishing junior year was a major relief. My growing belly was just starting to make my school uniforms feel too small. I didn't worry about needing new uniforms though. My parents had made it clear that I wouldn't be returning to school. My teachers made it clear that girls who get pregnant don't go to college or do anything productive with their lives. So, I finished the year with the assumption that this would be my final experience in school forever.

Now, the summer felt easier for me. With the exception of time I spent at work, I could stay inside and avoid interactions with people. Simple trips to the grocery store or other places would start to make me feel uncomfortable. I'd bump into people I knew, or friends' parents who heard the news. Regardless, I would get stares from adults and comments from cashiers. Questions about my age, if I knew who the father was, if the father was involved, if I knew about condoms, why I hadn't been more responsible.

Engaging socially felt more exhausting as the days passed. And now, without my parents or my daughter's father, I relied mostly on my few friends and "A Baby Story" on TLC to keep me company. Watching that show was hard because so many of these moms felt support from someone during their pregnancies. They loved their growing bellies. Some talked about the challenges of trying to get pregnant. But I genuinely struggled to fall in love with my growing belly, as media would lead me to think I would.

Once I was able to get my own health insurance and get back into my prenatal appointments, I went to a clinic specifically for young moms. The waiting room's seats filled with other young women, sometimes with their partners or mothers. The nurse practitioner who saw me during each appointment treated me kindly and diligently did her best to help me understand the changes happening to my body.

But there were so many things changing outside of my body that I couldn't understand. Why were people treating me differently? Why were people making assumptions about my life? Who decided that young moms were destined for failure? And why and how had this become the dominant narrative?

But as my belly grew, something else changed too. The closer I got to meeting my baby, the more I started thinking about what kind of mother I wanted to be and what kind of life I wanted her to have. I thought about my education and how easy it is for me to thrive in school. Less than a week before the start of senior year, I went to the local school office and registered myself for a new – public – school. Now 6 months pregnant, I was determined to complete my senior year and graduate on time.

When I returned to school that Fall, I expected to face challenges. After getting my courses on the first week of school, I noticed my guidance counselor hadn't put me into any honors classes, although I had been in honors classes at my old school. I went back to her office and asked if that was a mistake. Surprised, she told me that this was because it was unlikely I'd graduate from high school, so didn't need to be in honors classes and I could just do what I could to get by in the other classes.

For the first few weeks, I easily aced every assignment and test. I grew impatient and disinterested in each one. Three of my seven teachers pulled me aside to tell me that it was clear I didn't belong there and should've been put in honors. When I explained what happened, one teacher connected me to a woman who would become my Title IX advocate. We walked back into the guidance counselor's office and explained that I needed to be put back into honors. Angry that I made a big fuss about it, she changed the schedule and sent me off with a sarcastic "good luck!" But I knew I didn't need it.

The coursework was easy and despite having horrible morning sickness for most of my pregnancy, I never fell behind. This infuriated a few of my teachers who didn't want me in their classes. At times, my teachers would humiliate me in front of class. They'd use me as an example when they wanted to remind others about failure, they would compare pregnant students' work to each other to see which one of us was slacking more than the others, and they'd shame me in front of class when it took me more than 4 min to waddle through a crowded building and 4 flights of stairs. The better I did in school, the harder they made it for me emotionally.

A few months later, when I returned to ask my counselor for help with my college application, she told me that I should focus on finishing high school first before thinking about college. She then pointed to a stack of community college brochures and told me those were my best options. At this point, I was exhausted. A part of me wanted to give up because it wasn't just in school but everywhere that I was surrounded by negativity.

Outside of school, I had horrible experiences in trying to access any sort of social assistance. Adult gatekeepers who were responsible for disseminating resources to people like me frequently made assumptions about my ability to make choices.

They seemed to believe that because I was pregnant and young, I must be lectured whenever possible on what was best for my child.

Despite all this, I found ways to make things work and excelled in school every day. Despite my exhaustion and pain and fear of what was to come, I was fully present in school each day until the days before I went into labor.

My daughter's father returned only 2 days before I went into labor. At the hospital, he stood by my head holding my hand while I cried in pain. After 19 h of labor and 25 min of pushing, my daughter was placed on my chest. I cried in a way I never did before. It was out of love, but also out of fear. I spent my whole pregnancy hearing that a child would ruin my life, so I wondered what this would mean for us.

Without anesthesia or any pain medication, the doctor began giving me stitches. I yelled from the pain, feeling every pinch and tug. She shushed me and told me it couldn't be worse than what I had just experienced and continued. Shortly after, a nurse asked me if I had started thinking about which birth control I wanted. Still in a daze from the lack of sleep and labor and delivery, I sat shocked at the question.

Two weeks later, I went back for a follow-up visit to make sure I was healing properly. At the appointment, a nurse asked me if I picked birth control yet. I hadn't. She recommended that I get Depo-Provera, I told her I'd think about it and pick something at my next appointment. Disappointed, she lectured me about the likelihood that I'd end up pregnant and back in her office in a few weeks if I didn't just get the depo shot. Exhausted, I said fine. She returned shortly after with the shot and sent me on my way.

Truthfully, I never wanted to have sex again. My body went through hell and my daughter's father and I weren't getting along. But on that day, it didn't matter. All that mattered to that nurse was that a girl like me didn't return in 3 months with another pregnancy. Yet, this was just another example of the ways in which I remained out of control over my own body–even after having a child.

During my maternity leave, the school was required to provide me with a tutor, but the tutor was only required to help me with 4 of my 7 classes. The school's vague policy left much up to the school's discretion. This meant they would put me in a position to fail 3 out of 7 classes that semester. When I complained to my school, they told me they had no obligation to help me beyond the minimum requirement.

I was lucky in one way. My psychology teacher signed up to be my tutor. Three days a week, she came to my house to check on my schoolwork, give me quizzes and tests, and hold my baby while I completed essays. Occasionally, we'd talk about motherhood and life. Never once did she make me feel inferior. She was the only person to remind me that regardless of age, motherhood is hard. It's harder when you're doing it alone. And even harder when you're young and being judged all the time. She went beyond the school's requirement and found ways to bring me quizzes and assignments for all of my classes so I wouldn't fail any. Because of her, I went back to school 6 weeks after my baby was born and was caught up in all of my classes.

Another challenge in school was my decision to exclusively breastfeed. When I requested a space to pump breastmilk twice a day, they told me that I was being difficult, looking for excuses to skip class, and should be using formula anyway. One of my teachers refused to let me leave class to pump milk and told me I needed to plan this around her class. On one specific occasion, I told her I couldn't wait until the end of class and needed to go pump. She denied this request. Towards the end of the class, my breasts began to leak milk through my shirt. In front of the class, she told me that I was leaking and should leave class. I was horrified and angry. Similarly, teachers wouldn't excuse medical absences for my daughter's appointments. She was born with congenital hypothyroidism, diagnosed at 5 days, and required weekly visits to have her blood drawn. Some teachers refused to accept excused absences for the days I took my daughter to the hospital saying, "You don't really need to go to the hospital that often."

I constantly felt like people around me were hoping for me to fail and doing anything they could to block my ability to make choices that would improve me and my child's future. It felt like it was more important to maintain a person like me as a stereotype than to say yes when I asked for some support. I realized that helping me not become a statistic was never in their plans.

I fought my school for the right to pump breastmilk and won, I challenged teachers who violated my Title IX rights and won, and I walked the stage with my graduating high school class with my 6-month-old daughter in the crowd.

The journey after high school wasn't easy either. My daughter's father would often disappear, my relationship with my parents was broken, and I had lost connections to the people who previously cared about me. It very much felt like it was just my daughter and me pushing against the world to just live a normal happy life. But I was strongly motivated to make something of myself so that my daughter would go to be so proud of me. I often thought about the kinds of stories I'd hope my daughter could tell her grandchildren about me or the kind of legacy I could leave behind for them. I thought about how my experiences could end with me and that I could work to both improve our lives while changing the environment around us.

It meant removing myself from people who felt like toxic influences, frequently trying to convince me that I would end up unhappy and in poverty no matter how hard I tried to fight it. There were so many times when I wondered if the things these people were saying were true. What if I was destined for failure? What if everything I'm trying to change can't be changed?

There were many things I didn't know, but I did know that I wanted to try for my daughter. I spent years in and out of college trying to take my time to work towards a degree that would advance my career. I worked in healthcare, nonprofit, then went on to co-found an organization by and for young moms. Later, I was recruited to join a tech company in Silicon Valley to bring my expertise learned on the job and from life and leadership into a new sector.

The expectations for girls like me is that we don't finish high school, go to college, or become good mothers. The expectations are defined by stereotypes and our motivation stifled by shame. But I knew that I had two options: let society define my future or define it for myself. I chose the latter.

A few years ago, I went back to Brazil to spend time with family. I realized that cultural attitudes there are very different from what I experienced in the USA, and it's possible for a culture to be supportive of young mothers. While there, I asked my cousins, aunts, and uncles about the young mothers in our families. The first thing they all said was that in Brazil, you are a simply a mother, and not labeled as a "young mother" or "teen mother." Culturally, no one refers to the mothers in their families as young mothers.

The next thing they told me was that there were so many young mothers in our family that it would be easier to name those who were not young. But they couldn't understand where the line was drawn between "young" and no longer young. Who would define that?

Lastly, they pointed out that in a country where sex education is terrible, access to birth control and condoms is a challenge, abortion is illegal, and the government restricts women's autonomy over their own bodies, there are bound to be lots of unplanned pregnancies. And when it happens, there's nothing you can do at the point but prepare for parenthood. The regret, disbelief, or anger that one might feel about an unplanned pregnancy all remain valid reactions, but when you have no options, you have no choice, literally, but to force yourself to move on. And peers and family members move on too.

Also, in Brazil, where families often have deep roots in the community, the neighbors gather to offer support and resources to a family as a whole when somebody is ill or when somebody is pregnant. Helping each other is a vital part of survival.

Their beautiful description of the world they live in made me feel sick knowing that my parents moved 5000 miles away for a better life, yet their own daughter and granddaughter would face a stigma that doesn't exist where they came from. While it made me wonder if our lives could've been better if my pregnancy occurred in Brazil, I still held on to the reality that, despite my teenage pregnancy, I still did go on to do what most immigrants and Americans alike dream of doing.

After my negative experiences within the education system, I forced myself to spend more time learning at home. Full of energy in my early 20s, I traded hours of sleep for online courses. Anything I could learn, I tried it and I took time to learn whatever I needed to compensate for what others would assume I lacked. I dedicated myself to understanding the intricacies of rapidly developing new technologies like social media so I could gain expertise that my peers lacked. I found gaps and I filled them, trying to both prove my worth and maintain my role as a valuable member of the time. More importantly, my ability to overcome personal struggles helped me see all struggles as temporary. That it was never a matter of if I could overcome a challenge, but how. The mentality of having been a teenage mom who changed the odds gave me the courage I needed to do it in every part of my identity.

By 25, I was working at the Brigham and Women's Hospital on their health equity team and training people across the city on how to use new technologies. By 27, I was recruited by an ex-Googler in Silicon Valley to help build a tech startup. In an industry where less than 3% of women are Latina, it made me so proud to not just be Latina, but a young Latina mother in this space. And by the age of 11, my daughter learned how to code and build video games, participating in competitions at MIT.

I know that these are important accomplishments, but I also know my daughter's and my biggest accomplishments will never be as visible as professional roles or materialistic output.

Despite society's assumptions, my daughter's birth is what prompted me to think more deeply about the person I want to become and the impact I want to make on the world around us. Although my role is to raise her and teach her what I know, the experience of being a mother also taught me a lot about myself, my ability to overcome, and created an expectation for myself that is solely based on growing. We teach each other the language and agency we need to have complete control over our lives. And my desire to give her a better life propelled me into a several year journey in therapy to work on trauma, PTSD, and anxiety so I could be healthier and happier.

Today, the proudest part of my story is that my daughter and I have the power to define our lives and our stories. We have the language and the agency to have complete control over our bodies. We feel safe, we experience happiness, and we get to explore life outside the stereotypes that were expected of us. With her, I don't feel alone in this journey and that has enabled us both to thrive.

Anna's Story: An Intergenerational Cycle

I found out 4 months after my 16th birthday that I was pregnant. Shortly after came the morning sickness, only it was ALL day long. My doctor sent me for an ultrasound because he was concerned about my feeling so sick. That's when I found out I was having TWINS! I was terrified. I was going to be a mom of 2 babies in just a few months and hadn't even finished high school. I knew no matter what from the day I found out that there was only one option, to keep my baby/babies and that never changed. My sister had become pregnant at 16 and had an abortion, then later had her first daughter at 19. I could never do that. My mom was very supportive, although hurt and shocked, but she too had become a mom at 18. My grandparents were disappointed to say the least but still stayed supportive for the most part.

The second blow for my family was finding out that not only was I pregnant but by a black man, which in their day wasn't heard of and definitely not accepted. It took some time but that eventually passed and was accepted also.

My great aunt came to visit from Colorado when I was 6–7 months along and tried to convince me to move to Denver to a home where I would live with other teen mothers and give my babies up for adoption. She said that I was selfish, and that it was unfair to everyone else. She argued that my mom would end up raising them and that they would never have a chance. She also pointed out that they would be ridiculed for being biracial by both Blacks and Whites, and that I would be nothing and basically so would they.

Being pregnant in general was rough, especially when not only was I 16 but I looked 12. I got many stares (especially from elderly people) and was told by my boyfriend's mother the first time I met her not to expect him to stay with me just because I was pregnant. We didn't really ever get along after that.

I delivered my son and daughter via scheduled C-section 2 weeks before my due date and they were both healthy at 6 pounds and 20 inches each! I was over the moon in love and beyond ecstatic after being such a high-risk pregnancy. We stayed in the hospital 3 days and went home to start our lives. I lived with my mom still, seeing as how I turned 17 two days before they were born, and my boyfriend ended up staying to help. It was supposed to be temporary but became permanent. Even though my mom didn't like it, I needed the help.

I finished school that year from home and went back to high school for my senior year. I was able to go to school half a day and work half a day. I completed my senior year and graduated with my 2 beautiful babies in the audience. When I was 18 my boyfriend and I moved out and into our first house – a rental – for our little family and married 2 years later. The marriage only lasted 5 years. Sadly, he was unfaithful throughout our entire relationship. From day one, I knew he was unfaithful, but I wouldn't give up, especially now that we had children. It wasn't until one day when I realized my focus had switched from my kids, and instead to catching him being unfaithful, that I stopped and asked myself what I was doing. The next day I told him I wanted a divorce. After that it was a long year of fighting and court dates, emotions, you name it. I was also diagnosed and hospitalized for Crohn's disease during this time and was told I shouldn't have been alive. I vowed to never give up and I would fight to get better. A couple years after the divorce, my ex stopped paying child support and I was left to do it all alone. I did. I did everything both parents would do. My kids graduated from high school, went to college and are now 23 years old. My daughter is an RN and my son is in his last year of college. I couldn't be prouder of them and the choice I made 23 years ago. It was never an easy road and still isn't, but we made it.

Elizabeth's Story: On Being the Child of a Teen Mother

My mother, Melissa, was 16 years old when I was born. For the first 5 years of my life I lived with her, my two grandparents, and my uncle who was 18 years old and an aunt who was 13 when I was born. I have many fond memories from that time. It was a different life from what was yet to come. I remember running around the house hurtling over toys and sliding on the kitchen floor. I grew very close to my grandparents in a way that I can only assume mimics the bond one would have with their biological parents. My grandmother took the primary caregiving role, so my mother and I developed more like sisters than mother and daughter. I felt that I had a secure home.

When I was five, my mother and I moved out to live with her new boyfriend, who became the father of my half brother and sister. After leaving my grandparent's home, my life became a series of unfortunate events. To begin with, it was heart wrenching to be taken from my family and the people I considered my parents. No one understood why I was struggling to cope with this separation, which led to a lot of acting out, with the result that I was often punished. This alienated me from my mother, who I imagine interpreted my behavior as evidence I didn't like her, and alienated her from me. I'm not sure if at 20 years of age I would have reacted differently and been able to understand the difference between my child's missing their old environment and her not "liking" me. This divide has never truly mended, and I often wonder if the lack of initial bonding contributed to it.

Due to my mother's lack of resources, low education level, and lack of maturity; she tended to have poor decision-making skills, with the result that we were often in bad circumstances. She struggled to find work that was over minimum wage, despite graduating from high school. My then stepfather was verbally abusive at best and had isolated her from her family, cutting us off from what could have been a source of support. Before I was able to start financially contributing to the family, we lived in severe poverty; at one point living in a tent for six months. During that time, I distinctly remember learning a valuable lesson on what "water resistant" means. Lying between my siblings and the side of the tent, during a particularly scary storm, I was soaked by the rain coming in through the tent walls. I remember the pain of the cold water and the tent slapping across my legs and back. I still get a painful sensation when splashed with cold water.

Additionally, we spent many days hungry and not knowing where we would sleep that night. My mother developed what I now recognize was major depressive disorder. These episodes began when I was roughly 10 years old. I made sure my younger siblings were fed, dressed, and made it to the school bus, while also attempting to get myself ready for school as well. I remember being bullied for the tattered clothes and shoes with holes I had to wear, because we didn't have the money to replace them. I often fantasized about what my life would had been like if I were living with my grandparents. My mother, despite trying as hard as she could, was never able treat me as a child rather than a sibling. This I think is partly because she had to rely on me for so much, and partly due to the lost early bonding time. Even today she will slip and call me her sister or refer to my grandmother as "our mom."

Throughout these years my stepfather was frequently absent. He had a habit of moving us to different locations and disappearing for months at a time. I can remember being evicted from no less than seven homes. One time when I was twelve I broke down in the doorway because the landlord informed me we had 30 days to move. I went to more than seven schools before I was in sixth grade, being at one school only 3 months. This constant isolation caused a significant decrease in the amount of time I had with my grandparents. From the time I was in second grade until we returned to Oklahoma prior to starting my sixth grade year, I only saw my grandparents once every year or two years. Despite the distance, I still felt deeply loved by my grandparents and grieved every time we had to leave.

One of the happiest days of childhood after leaving my grandparent's home, was during the summer of my 6th grade year. My stepfather had left the family to work overseas in an oilfield. The months leading up to that day were some of the darkest. We were abandoned in a small town in Texas. My mother did not have a job and we were struggling to get money for groceries. Many times, he would go weeks without contacting her and we finally heard the knock on the door from the landlord telling us to leave. Throughout these months, my mother was so depressed she would not leave the couch. She just laid there, barely speaking to any of us, staring into the distance. I made sure my sister and brother were fed and tried to take care of their basic needs the best a 12-year-old child possibly could.

But then, my grandfather came to get us. It's hard not to embellish the image I have of my grandfather pulling down the street with his horse trailer in tow. It was such a wonderful feeling to think I was getting to go back "home." I still remember having to be his side-view mirror, because he was missing one on the passenger side of his truck. It was like a rescue mission. I was so thankful and was so full of hope on that day.

When we got back to Oklahoma, we were living in a three-bedroom single wide trailer with my aunt and her two children, my uncle, and our family of four. It was cramped, but it felt nice being back with the people I had missed for so long. I remember many squabbles between myself and the other children in the household. Being the oldest by five-plus years, I had the unfortunate duty of babysitting everyone while my Aunt and Mother went to work. Even though this was a tough time, I have many happy memories of us all being together.

Then what seemed like a nightmare happened. After 2 years of happiness, my mother allowed my stepfather back into the family. Due to the cramped living situation, they decided to buy a home. How this occurred, I'm not completely sure. I can't imagine they had good credit with the number of evictions we had experienced and regularly not being able to pay bills. Once we moved into the home, things went back to being terrible. This was magnified by my being an adolescent and my stepfather making not so subtle advances towards me. So, I became angry at everyone. I was angry at my mother for taking him back, I was angry at everyone around me for not seeing his behavior, and I was angry at myself for being to scared to speak up. I know now I had no control over the situation and being a child at the time had no control over the behavior of the adults around me. However, at that time all I could feel was anger. This anger severed the parental bond which was once so strong between my grandparents and myself. I could not understand why they didn't fight harder to save me.

Despite the nightmare I lived at home, there was one place I felt safe and able to be the person I wanted to be; it was school. My love affair with school started in elementary school, although in an unlikely place. I remember standing in the line at the grocery store. I was so excited as the checker rang up the cart full of groceries, as we hadn't had anything to eat for several days. Once the food was all bagged in the cart to go, my mother wrote a check. Because of the amount, the cashier had to get a manager. I then remember watching as the grocery cart was pushed away by the man who'd been previously bagging them, because the manager said they would not accept checks from my mother any longer. I'm not sure the reason why, I can imagine the money wasn't there and it wasn't the first time out of desperation she wrote a hot check to feed her three children. As I sat in the back of my mother's car holding my crying little brother and sister with that gnawing pain throbbing in my stomach; I decided no matter what I would never let my future children live like this.

That moment was pivotal for me, and I'm very thankful for that moment. Because when times were very hard and my teenage brain encouraged me to do many reckless behaviors; I had a clear boundary of if it would impede my future it was a no go. This kept me away from drugs and terrified of pregnancy. I excelled at school, constantly winning awards, joined every extracurricular activity I could afford to be a part off, and played any sport that didn't require a lot of money to participate in. It was like having two lives, and school was the one that kept me safe. This become somewhat difficult by the end of my senior year, as we were evicted from our home once again. I couch surfed between several of my friends' until I could move into dorms on campus.

The road through college was tough. I worked 40-hour weeks while attempting full-time school. During holiday and school breaks I'd live in my car, as the dorms were closed during those times. Unfortunately, due to these circumstances I struggled to make the grades I needed to get into medical school. I had always dreamed of being a doctor but wasn't aware of the financial consequences of choosing such a path. I changed majors and taught in a local public school for four years; all the while working on my master's degree to improve my chances of being accepted to medical school. Eventually, I was accepted and chose a field that would allow me to work with high-risk children and provide hope to those who have had similar struggles.

My experiences are what made me the person I am today. They taught me to be resilient, how to hone my social skills, and how able to make friends from many demographics. It made getting an education a must and not a choice. It gave me a clear understanding of the consequences of falling short of my goals. Most importantly of all, it has taught me to be humble, thankful, and empathetic in a way I can't imagine learning without these trials.

I look back at the things my mother experienced and can't imagine being faced with those decisions in my late teens and early 20s. I truly believe her young age and lack of higher education made her vulnerable to manipulation and abuse. I also believe she faced a lot of stigma and discrimination in the workforce due to her being a young uneducated mother. All of these difficulties were probably factors in her becoming depressed to begin with and then compounded her depression. Stigma made her less likely to seek help.

In spite of all these obstacles, my mother has worked hard to reach a level of stability in her life. At the age of 50, she is still making far less than her classmates who had the opportunity to go further in their education. She has no retirement savings, and I worry about what will happen as she ages. She continues to have a very immature way of looking at the world and struggles with problem solving. We continue to have a sibling relationship; which has left me feeling orphaned in many ways due to the distance placed between myself and my grandparents.

As a new mother, I can't imagine trying to raise three children with no resources or support. When my first child was born, I was the same age as my grandmother when I was born. My grandmother was a teen mother herself, and I'm thankful I broke the cycle that seemed to plague my family. I've watched these women get left behind by society because of being so young when they began having children. My grandmother was forced to drop out of school because of her teen pregnancy. Some of these situations were a mark of their times, however, I have no doubt that teen mothers today face many of the same struggles and live with the same types of discrimination.

If I could send a message to teen mothers, it would be that there are people out there that want to help. It can be scary and hard to be a mother no matter what the age, and it does not mean you're not a good mother. Despite what society may be telling you, your baby is not doomed to live in poverty and struggle. You still have many things to contribute to the world. I hope you find my story one of hope; as I feel like it made me better for it.

Discussion

There are really four stories here. Three involve teenage mothers (Natasha, and Anna and Melissa) and the fourth is the story of Melissa's child Elizabeth.

Natasha was stigmatized from the moment her pregnancy became known. Her parents forced her to move out, canceled her health insurance, and discontinued paying for private school. Her Catholic school seemed more concerned about dissuading her from having an abortion than giving her any support. On her own, she got medical insurance and enrolled in public school, graduating on time.

Natasha's experience with healthcare system when she attended a special clinic for young mothers was one of the few positive experiences she had with other people during her pregnancy. But the delivery was another story, which illustrates the punitive attitudes and disrespect which young women are often subjected to. The focus of her follow-up visit after the birth of her child was to keep her from having another child, not to engage her in a process of joint decision-making or encourage her to be a partner in her healthcare decisions.

After the birth of her child, Natasha's school offered little to her in the way of help or support, with the exception of one teacher who came to her home and tutored her. When she returned to school she was subjected to harassment. Although she was a good student, she had to fight to get into honors classes, and the school discouraged her from even thinking of applying to college.

Eventually Natasha's parents accepted her. She went on to develop a career for herself in technology, basically educating herself. She herself became a passionate advocate against the stigma that young parents face, working with an advocacy group for young parents. Both she and her daughter are thriving. She takes pride in having overcome many obstacles, and having gone from feeling she had no control over her life to having a sense of agency and imparting this to her daughter.

Natasha's story is also one of intersectionality, that of being an immigrant and Latina as well as a young mother. She describes the cultural differences between her country of origin, Brazil, and the US. We can speculate how these differences may have led to difficulties negotiating adolescence. She also experienced sexual abuse, exposure to domestic violence, and depression, all known risk factors for teen pregnancy. She describes how these adverse experiences reduced her sense of control and agency, to the point that she "stopped caring what would happen" to her.

Anna described getting support from her family despite their disapproval of her pregnancy. We know this is a fairly common trajectory. Her boyfriend also offered support in the beginning, as did the man whom she later married. She was able to complete school, participating in a work-study program, and her family provided childcare to allow her to do this. Her main problems were a difficult high-risk pregnancy and the stigma she experienced from strangers. Unlike Natasha who was threatened with eternal damnation, she was pressured to have an abortion.

Anna describes how people stared at her when she was pregnant. How a relative tried to convince her to have an abortion, telling her she and her children would be doomed to failure if she did not. Like Natasha's her situation is intersectional, combining the stigma of an interracial relationship with that of a teen pregnancy.

Although we don't hear directly from Elizabeth's mother Melissa, we have a sense of what her life must have been like. Her own mother had been a teenage mother and dropped out of school. At first, she ceded child-rearing responsibilities to her mother; although this meant a secure attachment for Elizabeth, it doesn't seem to have increased Melissa's ability to function independently. Melissa attempted to provide a life for herself and her children; she must have hoped the future would be brighter than it turned out to be. At first, she, her baby, and the father of her child lived with her parents; later she moved out and married another man. As is the case with many young parents, it didn't work out. The marriage failed despite Melissa's persistence and willingness to accept her husband's infidelity for a period of time. She and her children lived in poverty and unstable conditions. Her relationship with the daughter who was born to her when she was 16 (Elizabeth) was strained from the time she attempted to take over the responsibilities of parenthood from her parents. The stresses of poverty and marital problems, plus the challenge of parenting her daughter whose early bonding was to her grandparents, set them both up for failure. There were economic as well as emotional costs for both Melissa, who did not complete her education and has worked at low paying jobs. She has worked hard and survived but not thrived.

Elizabeth describes many typical experiences of children of teen parents. Some are directly related to the difficulty of some young mothers in providing adequate parenting (being "good enough mothers"), and others are grounded in psychosocial adversity: poverty, homelessness, multiple school changes, and stigma. In contrast to her mother, she overcame the odds and has done well.

Each of these stories is a tale of resilience in the face of stigma. We see how stigma impacts its victims by becoming internalized; in Natasha's words "There were so many times when I wondered if the things these people were saying were true."

None of these young women who became mothers planned their pregnancies. They certainly do not fit the stereotype that a lack of personal responsibility and the lure of financial support through the welfare system were responsible for their pregnancies. None of their families were pleased about the pregnancy and in one case, reacted extremely negatively. In three cases, the young mothers had mothers who themselves had their first children as teenagers. This is not uncommon [2]. Their stories confirm what we have known for a long time about the link between psychosocial adversity and teen pregnancy [1].

While one could argue that had these young women been better informed about the risks of unprotected sex and had access to reproductive health care in their schools or communities, their pregnancies would not have occurred, the fact is that they did. What they experienced after they became pregnant is at least as important as what happened before. Basically, they were told they would never amount to anything. The only support they received was from their own families, and even this was not unconditional. Outside they experienced stigma – when out in public with their children, at school. The stigma they and their children experienced made positive outcomes unlikely. Remarkably, they and their children managed to survive all this and even when they continued to struggle, were able to support their children.

Somehow, they were propelled by reservoirs of strength that they found within themselves, with little support from outside. Hearing their stories, one wonders how this happened.

Natasha summarizes it well:

> The expectations for girls like me are that we don't finish high school, go to college, or become good mothers. The expectations are defined by stereotypes and our motivation stifled by shame. But I knew that I had two options: let society define my future or define it for myself. I chose the latter.

As we demonstrate in the following chapters, the research evidence provides support for such good outcomes in many cases, as young parents marshal their strengths, develop a sense of pride in themselves and their accomplishments, become productive members of society, and provide excellent parenting to their children. How much easier would it have been if they had been given essential support and encouragement along the way?

References

1. Hillis SD, Anda RF, Dube SR, Felitti VJ, Marchbanks PA, Marks JS. The association between adverse childhood experiences and adolescent pregnancy, long-term psychosocial consequences, and fetal death. Pediatrics. 2004;113(2):320–7.
2. Meade CS, Kershaw TS, Ickovics JR. The intergenerational cycle of teenage motherhood: an ecological approach. Health Psychol. 2008;27(4):419–29.

Stigma and Its Consequences for Adolescent Mothers and Their Babies

3

Jean-Victor P. Wittenberg

Introduction

Social stigma occurs in all social groups. It serves to reinforce power differentials, protecting the advantages of one group and marginalizing stigmatized groups. It has profound effects on the lives on those who are stigmatized. Pregnant teens and teen parents are clearly exposed to stigma. Expressions of social stigma directly harm these young mothers and their babies. This chapter reviews evidence of stigmatizing attitudes toward teen pregnancy. It explores how stigma contributes to social disadvantage and increases the risk of teens becoming pregnant. It examines the multiple ways in which stigma contributes to many of the negative outcomes of teen pregnancy for both mothers and their babies. We are convinced that stigma is a significant predictor of adverse outcomes for many teens and their babies and that many would do better were it not for the impact of social disapprobation.

Social Stigma and Teen Pregnancy

Adolescent girls from the ages of 15–19 years are usually the focus in the literature on teen pregnancy. Pregnancy does occur in younger girls but at a lower rate and is usually excluded from surveys and studies. Teen pregnancy, previously out-of-wedlock pregnancy, has long carried a social stigma. In the past a greater proportion of adolescents who became pregnant were married; they may have suffered less stigma [26]. Although there are some reports that stigma does not impact adolescent mothers in some parts of the world many other publications indicate that stigma against teen mothers is globally pervasive and very damaging (e.g., a WHO report

J.-V. P. Wittenberg (✉)
University of Toronto, Toronto, ON, Canada

Hospital for Sick Children, Toronto, ON, Canada
e-mail: jean.wittenberg@sickkids.ca

J.-V. P. Wittenberg et al. (eds.), *Adolescent Pregnancy and Parenting*,
https://doi.org/10.1007/978-3-031-42502-8_3

from February 2018, https://www.who.int/news-room/fact-sheets/detail/adolescent-pregnancy). Stigma has been demonstrated to be associated with exclusion from education, health, and social resources, even with mortality. Adolescent pregnancy is the leading cause of death for girls aged 15–19 globally [40].

Stigma related to teen pregnancy has been pervasive in the USA for many years; social disapproval of out-of-wedlock births was very strong in the early Puritan settlements. Page [31] wrote that stigma has discriminated against unmarried mothers for two main reasons: their sexual activity elicited disapproval from the Christian church and secondly, secular authorities disapproved of what they saw as "the 'blameworthy' public dependency of this group." Ironically some teen mothers become more productive members of their communities [26, 33] but that finding is obscured by the social bias.

To understand sexual activity and mores in the Puritan age, Thompson [35] studied court records from Middlesex County, which covered a large area of the Massachusetts Bay Colony in the seventeenth century. Laws prohibited fornication (sex between unmarried individuals) and adultery and provided for punishment by whipping (up to 20 lashes) and fines. Out-of-wedlock birth, or a full-term birth that occurred prior to 9 months after marriage, was presumptive evidence of fornication. Midwives were tasked with reporting cases. Male and female perpetrators were held equally culpable. Women were obliged to reveal the identity of the father. Revelations made to a midwife while a woman was in labor carried heavy weight. She might lose the assistance of the midwife. She might fear having to face heaven's wrath if she lied. Fathers (or those judged to be the fathers by the court in cases of contested paternity) had to pay for the support of the child. This draconian approach was based on the towns' fiduciary interest in not having to be financially responsible for children born outside of marriage, in addition to their adherence to Puritan morality. In addition to the opprobrium meted out to individual sinners, the whole town was held responsible for any moral failures of its inhabitants and faced potential punishment from God if they did not act decisively.

Thompson calculated from the court records that teen premarital pregnancy was quite rare—with an incidence of only about 0.5% of the population (much lower than that in England at the time) but he also found evidence that pregnant women resorted to abortion, infanticide, or fleeing the area, so the actual incidence was probably considerably higher. He concluded that premarital sex was certainly not unknown among teenagers in the area, most of whom did not marry until their mid-twenties. Regardless of the actual prevalence of teen pregnancy, the existence of very punitive attitudes is undeniable, and suggests a continuity between seventeenth century attitudes of condemnation and the stigma that persists today.

There is a strong belief in professional, political, and public sectors that having a baby in adolescence blights the lives of teen-aged girls. These beliefs persist even though some studies that examine the long-term trajectory of young women's lives suggest that for many women having a baby in adolescence is not a roadblock to development, and in fact may have spurred a more adaptive and constructive posture and led to better outcomes when compared to their socioeconomic peers. We review this literature in Chap. 4. This ironic finding, that some adolescent girls find better life trajectories because of pregnancy, must also be understood in the context of their finding ways to overcome negative social attitudes, i.e., stigma, which operated prior to their pregnancies and continues after their baby is born.

Stigma and How It Operates

In its earliest usage stigma refers to some form of mark or stain; it derives from a Greek word denoting a brand burned into the skin of individuals to show that they were criminals or runaway slaves [30]. In the present day the term has been used to refer to physical appearance, conduct or ethnicity that are seen as inferior [31]. Stigma has often been identified as a problem for people with mental health disorders, both in the past and in the present.

Erving Goffman's [13] book *Stigma: Notes on the Management of Spoiled Identity* inspired an escalation of research on many aspects of stigma. This research has repeatedly demonstrated the negative impact of stigma on the lives of the stigmatized. He categorized stigma as targeting:

1. Physical health issues (e.g., HIV, mental health);
2. Association with marginalized groups (e.g., racial or ethnic identity);
3. Moral or behavioral characteristics (e.g., alcoholism, teen pregnancy).

Hatzenbuehler et al. [16] define stigma as the "co-occurrence of labeling, stereotyping, separation, status loss and discrimination in a context within which power is exercised." They conceptualize it as a fundamental social cause of health inequalities. In this it is very specifically relevant to the situation for teen mothers and their babies.

The mechanisms for how stigma operates are complex and interactive. Link and Phelan [22] conceptualized stigma as dynamic, a social process governed by political power based in social status and wealth. Those in power construct and impose ideals that lead to preferred and stigmatized social identities. These are then reflected in structural differences in society. Chambers and Erausquin [5] wrote: "There are multiple forms or manifestations of stigma: internalized stigma (i.e., the acceptance of negative attributes of one's own social identities), enacted stigma (i.e., experienced discrimination from a person based upon one's social identities), symbolic stigma (i.e., community norms towards discrimination of groups of people based upon their social identities), and structural stigma (i.e., establishment of discriminating laws and enforcement towards groups of people based upon their social identities). The different manifestations of stigma are important to consider when examining adolescent pregnancy and motherhood, since they suggest multiple ways in which stigma may shape attitudes, experiences, and behaviors" (p. 2).

Stigma can be applied to groups, and thus to the individual members of a group: for gender (e.g., female, transgender, gender nonconforming), social status (e.g., poor, welfare), race (e.g. Black), ethnicity (e.g. Latinx), immigrant status, religion (e.g. Jewish, Muslim), health (e.g. living with a disability, HIV), age (e.g. adolescent, senior), or conduct (e.g. criminal, sexually active adolescent). In each case the stigmatized group or individual is seen as inferior, undeserving, bad, or threatening. Often these groups or individuals are identified with multiple stigmatizing characteristics however, one label may be an outcome of another. For example, Black people in North America are more likely to be poor because of racist attitudes but the poverty is often attributed to be the result of individual or group inferiority. The same is often true of beliefs about pregnant or mothering teens. They are believed to be poor because they became pregnant. Well-controlled studies have shown that rather than being an outcome of pregnancy, poverty is a predictor of pregnancy. Furthermore, inequitable gender norms and social norms that condone violence against women put girls at greater risk of unintended pregnancy (https://www.who.int/news-room/fact-sheets/detail/adolescent-pregnancy).

Acceptance of one inaccurate premise leads to beliefs in many other inaccurate or untrue conclusions; for example, pregnant teens are promiscuous and exploitative. They are seen as a drain on the public purse; however, studies have shown that over the long term many of these young women become more productive and contributing members of their communities than their socioeconomic peers. (e.g., SmithBattle 2009).

Intersectional Stigma

Intersectional stigma is a concept that addresses the additive effects of multiple lines of discrimination focused on individuals or groups [36]. The term was coined by Black feminist scholars to describe how multiple kinds of stigma interact to compound negative impacts [8]. Thus, being a member of a minority group plus having HIV-AIDS, for example, multiplies the effects of stigma.

Grollman [14], for example, demonstrated that multiple forms of perceived discrimination have an additive effect on self-reported depressive symptoms and global assessment of physical health. Intersectional theory conceives of the different axes along which discrimination acts. These axes can act in tandem, interacting and leading to higher levels of oppression and to more rigid and prejudiced belief systems about groups and individuals within those groups. For example, poverty is seen as an undesirable and stigmatized characteristic. Teen pregnancy is characterized in the same way, however, what is not seen is that poor teens are more likely to become pregnant; rather they are more likely to be perceived as being poor because of their becoming pregnant. Both pregnancy and poverty are often perceived as self-inflicted, the results of low moral fiber; thus, they are targets for stigmatizing attitudes.

The Impact of Stigma

Stigma affects individuals in multiple, interacting, and accumulating ways—affecting health, development, and life opportunities. It is associated with undesirable health outcomes including poor mental health, physical health, academic underachievement, infant mortality, low social status, poverty, and reduced access to housing, education, and jobs [9, 13, 16, 25].

Stigma acts to discredit an individual or group of individuals [9, 13]. Persons who are stigmatized are devalued because they have some attribute that is believed by others to make them inferior, unworthy, or undesirable [9].

Social beliefs influence distribution of and accessibility to resources, which are central to the provision of opportunities for development and betterment. To a significant degree groups continue to hold beliefs that deprive stigmatized sectors of their societies from the opportunities they need to become respected and productive members of their communities. Beliefs that certain groups are undeserving, or inferior impede access to resources such as education and jobs, thereby contributing to poverty, which of course carries its own power to generate undesirable health outcomes.

Stigmatizing interactions foster the development of negative self-representations and low self-esteem. They lead to social isolation. Accepting the discrimination as fair, deserved and expectable is likely to lead to reduced efforts to do better, to reach higher.

Furthermore, the same characteristics that evoke stigma may be secondary to stigma. For example, those who are poorly educated or unemployed may be seen as inferior, but stigma also deprives them of educational and vocational opportunities, dooming them to continue living in poverty and continued stigmatization.

The impact of stigma is subtle and especially difficult to recognize by those who hold social power. Power differentials are central to the influence of stigma. Negative misattributions can be held by any individuals or groups towards others. When they are exercised by the individual or group that has power they have lasting and negative impacts. Stigma is effective because of the power of group beliefs against a weaker subgroup [16]. These beliefs provide advantages to the group in power. When power relationships are changed, outcomes are changed. For example, higher rates of depression in women vs. men are reduced when women have more power within a society [34].

Stigma and Social Media

Social media have become a powerful force influencing many people around the world. Social media have become powerful and influential conveyors of misinformation and disinformation; these are components of stigma. Adolescents and young adults are heavy users of social media [1, 29]. There are occasions in which it can have beneficial effects [2, 29]. Stigmatized individuals find friends and support online. Organizations use social media to support their advocacy efforts. Vehicles have included education, social communications, community involvement, collaborative projects and even in some circumstances advocacy against stigma associated with issues such as youth mental health (e.g. Headstrong [17]—a youth focused initiative to provide identification, respect and support for youth with mental health problems) or sexual discrimination (e.g., Healthy Teen Network [18] which focuses on teen's right to make their own sexual choices and decisions and their right to respect and support.) Much of the effect of social networks remains to be demonstrated empirically [1] but adverse uses are widely reported as well: social isolation, cyberbullying, online harassment, sexual solicitation, etc. These are associated with very serious consequences such as depression or even suicide especially in more vulnerable youth (Kelly et al. 2019; [24]). Challenges facing us include finding ways to accurately understand the impact of social media and to mitigate its adverse effects.

Stigmatization as a Risk Factor for Teen Pregnancy

Birth rates are highest among those young women who are socially and economically disadvantaged, such as being poor, belonging to a minority, being in the child protection system, or others [12, 26, 33]. These groups are already marginalized. They are more likely to become pregnant for many reasons, each young woman and her choices must be understood individually, and once pregnant are more likely to become targeted by stigma for multiple reasons.

Within disadvantaged groups there are characteristics that select for those girls who are more likely to become pregnant as teens. Those who have been exposed to violence [6], or who have psychiatric disorders [37], a history of maltreatment [12, 19, 28, 32], lack of education [20], and/or knowledge and access to contraception [21] are more likely to become pregnant. Among adolescents in care, pregnant or mothering teens are more likely than other young women in care to have engaged in more risky behavior, have been exposed to more forms of maltreatment, have fewer social supports, and to have more psychiatric symptoms [12]. Mollborn [26] refers to girls who are more likely to become pregnant as descending into "life worlds of chaos" even before becoming pregnant; for these girls' pregnancy and motherhood are outcomes of disorganization, disadvantage, and chaos.

There are also teens, who may be already in stigmatized groups or not, who choose to become pregnant or to keep a pregnancy. The validity of their choices is often dismissed, swept away by rigid, stigmatizing attitudes in others.

Attitudes of Health Care Professionals

Stigma influences the attitudes of healthcare professionals to teen mothers. Breheny and Stephens [4] analyzed transcripts of individual interviews with 17 New Zealand health professionals (doctors, midwives, and nurses) to examine the discourses used to construct adolescent motherhood. Their statements regarding adolescent mothers depicted them as naive, distracted, and self-centered, and hence unable to mother correctly. The professionals demonstrated beliefs about teens that conflicted with their seeing them as anything but incapable mothers. These attitudes, which may also have been influenced by the teens' belonging to other stigmatized groups, inevitably influence their interactions with teen mothers, who experience healthcare providers as dismissive, offensive, demeaning, or hurtful. Such stressful interactions are likely to discourage prenatal and post-natal care, as well as well-baby visits.

Influence on Research

Stigma influences even the construction and conclusions in research on pregnant adolescents. For example, many studies focus on links between teenage parenting and poverty, with the assumption that being a teen parent leads to poverty. As Bonell [3] pointed out:

> Many studies justified their interest in teenage pregnancy in terms of its effects on the poverty of parents and children. However, although these authors provided numerous examples of how teenage parenting could be accompanied by poverty, "none acknowledged that such poverty is not an inevitable consequence of teenage parenthood, but rather is mediated by the way society responds to the needs (and the potential) of teenagers and their children [3, p. 268].

More recent reviews (e.g., [26]) have illuminated the association that links pre-existing poverty to increased rates of adolescent pregnancy. Many earlier studies concluded that pregnancy led teens into poverty, but they used a more general, more advantaged comparison group rather than comparing to peers with equal disadvantage. In comparison to peers, mothering teens can do as well or better with regards to education, income, etc.

Young Mothers' Experiences

Stigma is a significant and frequent experience for many teen mothers, although it has not been as well studied as other kinds of stigma, such as stigma associated with mental illness or sexual orientation. An exploratory study of 925 low-income teen mothers in southeastern Texas retrospectively evaluated the mothers' experience of stigmatization during pregnancy within days of delivery; their self-reported ratings were then correlated with a variety of behavioral, social, and sociodemographic characteristics [39]. Thirty-nine per cent said they experienced social stigmatization during their pregnancies.

Regression analysis indicated that the following variables made independent contributions to the young mothers' perceptions of stigmatization: social isolation, lack of involvement with their baby's father, aspirations to complete college, Caucasian race, experiencing family criticism, fearing being hurt by other teenagers, and experiencing verbal abuse by family, partner, or peers. On the other hand, higher self-esteem and having dropped out of school were found to be protective against feeling stigmatized.

Although our ability to draw inferences from this study is limited by its having utilized a single self-report item to evaluate stigma, by its geographic homogeneity, and by its retrospective design, the work of these investigators is useful because it draws attention to the phenomenon of social stigmatization within the context of teen pregnancy and motherhood. The authors note that while, in the middle of that last century, pregnant adolescents we often removed from their own homes and communities—these teens and their pregnancies are now much more visible to family members, in school, and in the community. As a result, the consequences of social stigma may be more immediate in the experience of today's pregnant teenager.

Regardless of the actual experience of being stigmatized, individuals who are members of stigmatized groups can internalize the identity of the devalued group. "Self-stigmatization," a belief that negative stereotypes apply to oneself, has profound effects on self-image and identity, both key aspects of adolescent development [7]. Self-stigmatization is associated with the expectation of being devalued by others [23].

A Canadian study compared younger and older mothers with respect to their perceptions of stigmatization, using in-depth interviews [38]. Young mothers from Anglophone Euro-Canadian groups experienced the most stigma, noting that in play groups, on buses, and in a variety of other settings they sensed disapproval by others. The older mothers did not experience this. Those who were from communities where early childbearing was encouraged and considered normal did not generally experience stigma. There are differing attitudes to young motherhood. Research into outcomes for both the teen mothers and their children might help us understand more about the deleterious effects of this type of stress.

Stigma as a Source of Stress for Young Mothers

Stigma against pregnant and parenting teens operates at multiple levels—structurally in policy and regulatory systems, in social systems through sometimes unspoken but often overt communications, in interpersonal interactions when individuals or groups act on stigmatizing beliefs, and within individuals who have internalized stigmatized representations of themselves. Examples of operationalization of stigma at a structural level include exclusion from school and policies that prohibit excused absences for taking a child to medical appointments. Social stigma manifests in communications like those that occur in medical offices or schools that make medical treatment or education difficult or even impossible to achieve. Interpersonal stigma is manifested by behaviors of individuals toward the stigmatized person, such as the sneers that occur on the street. As we have seen in the case of Natasha (in Voices of Lived Experience), it might involve the refusal of a school counselor to write recommendations for college, and telling a student she should not even think about applying. Peer victimization, bullying, and harassment are also manifestations of interpersonal stigmatization. The National Women's Law Center's

[27] website contains the following examples, all of which are prohibited under US law:

- A student becomes pregnant, and now a group of girls are repeatedly texting her during class and tweeting about her at school, calling her a "slut" and a "whore."
- A girl becomes pregnant, and fellow students have been spreading rumors about her sexual behavior, repeatedly asking her questions about the "baby daddy," inquiring how many times she's had sex and what position she and her partner were in when she got pregnant, etc.
- A student who is pregnant has been repeatedly sexually propositioned by a group of boys in her class. They say things like, "we know you put out," and "why would a girl like you say no?"

Finally, at an individual level, stigma has profound psychological and physiological effects. It affects identity and sense of self, and may result in a sense of shame, loneliness and isolation, increased vigilance, and ruminative tendencies [38]. Social exclusion, a component of stigma, has been shown to impact cortisol levels [11]. It has been shown to be associated with increased blood pressure, and effects on the HPA axis [10] and with effects on cortisol in LGBTQ youth [15]. Stigma undoubtedly has adverse effects on the psychology, mental health, physical health, and day-to-day functioning for teen mothers.

Effects on Outcome

Social stigma is likely to play a key role in outcomes for both teens and their babies. Teens who belong to groups that are already stigmatized are at risk for further stigmatization when they become pregnant and then teen mothers. It is well-recognized that some adolescents who become pregnant and have babies have poorer outcomes than same age peers. These outcomes are largely predicted by factors that pre-existed the pregnancies. It is less often recognized that some teens who become pregnant significantly improve their life trajectories because of being young mothers [33].

Adolescents are in a vulnerable developmental phase in their lives. They are more likely than older individuals to fall prey to the more impulsive, less reflective decisions that are characteristic of their age. Impulsive decisions are more likely when teens are more stressed and less supported. Impulsive decisions affect not only the young mothers but also their babies. Even when young mothers find ways to improve their lives because of their taking on new childcare responsibilities, it may take time to reach a less stressful state. The teens may find themselves in a better position as time goes on, but their babies may have been exposed to what may be less than optimal experiences over the course of that time. Infants are particularly vulnerable because their early experiences become biologically embedded and influence them for the rest of their lives. Children born to young mothers struggle more than those born to older mothers. Stigma makes it worse; Zeiders et al. [41]

found that stigma in the first 2 years predicted maternal depression, insensitive maternal-child interactions, and lower child socio-emotional and academic performance at five years of age in a population of Mexican Americans in the USA. Further they found that the outcomes were related to the amount of discrimination and stress these families endured and that early childhood stresses in the first 3 years led to later difficulties.

Summary and Conclusions

Stigmatization has been shown to result in a variety of negative outcomes. Stigma and its consequences are compounded when teenage pregnancy or motherhood are added to pre-existing risk factors that are commonly found in this population. Stigmatization is potentially modifiable. To reduce or eradicate the adverse effects of stigma, power differentials must be addressed. Chambers and Erausquin [5] described strategies to reduce the negative health effects of stigma. These include empowerment to rebalance the power gradient inherent in in the process of stigma. Changing power gradients requires focusing on multiple societal levels to address how stigma develops and is perpetuated. Laws must be changed. Policies must be modified. Social and institutional attitudes must be recognized and modified. The goals are to encourage supportive responses from parents, physical and mental health service providers, educators, and social service personnel. At the individual level, some young mothers need individual support to cope with stigma and its psychological effects. Their babies and children need particular and specific interventions for developmental support as their mothers find their own ways to more fruitful and adaptive trajectories in their lives. We will discuss interventions to support and empower young parents in Chap. 7.

We are convinced that by informing social and professional attitudes and by addressing systemic bias we can change the stigma and stress that is imposed on teen mothers and their babies. We can significantly improve outcomes for teen mothers and their babies. Those changes are associated with important gains for the mothers and babies and for our communities.

References

1. Ahn J. The effect of social network sites on adolescents' social and academic development: current theories and controversies. J Am Soc Infor Sci Technol. 2011;62(8):1435–45.
2. Betton V, Borschmann R, Docherty M, Coleman S, Brown M, Henderson C. The role of social media in reducing stigma and discrimination. Br J Psychiatry. 2015;206(6):443–4.
3. Bonell C. Why is teenage pregnancy conceptualized as a social problem? A review of quantitative research from the USA and UK. Cult Health Sex. 2004;6(3):255–72.
4. Breheny M, Stephens C. Irreconcilable differences: health professionals' constructions of adolescence and motherhood. Soc Sci Med. 2007;64:112–24.
5. Chambers BD, Erausquin JT. The promise of intersectional stigma to understand the complexities of adolescent pregnancy and motherhood. J Child Adolesc Behav. 2015;3:1–5.

6. Copping LT, Campbell A, Muncer S. Violence, teenage pregnancy, and life history. Hum Nat. 2013;24(2):137–57.
7. Corrigan PW, Watson AC, Barr L. The self-stigma of mental illness: implications for self-esteem and self-efficacy. J Soc Clin Psychol. 2006;25(8):875–84.
8. Crenshaw KW. Demarginalizing the intersection of race and sex: a Black feminist critique of antidiscrimination doctrine, feminist theory, and antiracist politics. Univ Chic Leg Forum. 1989;139:139–67.
9. Crocker J, Major B, Steele C. Social stigma. In: Gilbert DT, Fiske ST, Lindzey G, editors. The handbook of social psychology. New York: McGraw-Hill; 1998. p. 504–53.
10. Dickerson SS, Kemeny ME. Acute stressors and cortisol responses. Psychol Bull. 2004;130(3):355–91. https://doi.org/10.1037/0033-2909.130.3.355.
11. Dickerson SS, Zoccola PM. Cortisol responses to social exclusion. In: The Oxford handbook of social exclusion. New York: Oxford University Press; 2013. p. 143–51.
12. Goodman D, Mazzuca A, Markle B, Cheung C, Titus A, Jellinek A. Partnerships for positive outcomes: Supporting young mothers in care. Children's Mental Health Ontario & Ontario Association for Children's Aid Societies Joint Conference; 2008.
13. Goffman E. Stigma. London: Penguin Books; 1963.
14. Grollman EA. Multiple forms of perceived discrimination and health among adolescents and young adults. J Health Soc Behav. 2012;53(2):199–214. https://doi.org/10.1177/0022146512444289.
15. Hatzenbuehler ML, McLaughlin KA. Structural stigma and hypothalamic–pituitary–adrenocortical axis reactivity in lesbian, gay, and bisexual young adults. Ann Behav Med. 2014;47(1):39–47.
16. Hatzenbuehler ML, Phelan JC, Link BG. Stigma as a fundamental cause of population health inequalities. Am J Public Health. 2013;103:813–21.
17. Headstrong. https://mentalhealthcommission.ca/training/headstrong/
18. Healthy Teen Network. https://www.healthyteennetwork.org/
19. Hillis SD, Anda RF, Dube SR, Felitti VJ, Marchbanks PA, Marks JS. The association between adverse childhood experiences and adolescent pregnancy, long-term psychosocial consequences, and fetal death. Pediatrics. 2004;113(2):320–7.
20. Imamura M, Tucker J, Hannaford P, da Silva MO, Astin M, Wyness L, et al. Factors associated with teenage pregnancy in the European Union countries: A systematic review. Eur J Public Health. 2007;17(6):630–6. https://doi.org/10.1093/eurpub/ckm014. Retrieved from http://www.ncbi.nlm.nih.gov/pubmed/17387106
21. Jozkowski KN, Crawford BL. The status of reproductive and sexual health in Southern USA: Policy recommendations for improving health outcomes. Sexuality Research & Social Policy: A Journal of the NSRC. 2016;13(3):252–62. https://doi.org/10.1007/s13178-015-0208-7.
22. Link BG, Phelan JC. Conceptualizing stigma. Annu Rev Sociol. 2001;27(1):363–85.
23. Link BG, Struening EL, Neese-Todd S, Asmussen S, Phelan JC. Stigma as a barrier to recovery: the consequences of stigma for the self-esteem of people with mental illnesses. Psychiatr Serv. 2001;52(12):1621–6.
24. Luxton DD, June JD, Fairall JM. Social media and suicide: a public health perspective. Am J Public Health. 2012;102(Suppl 2):S195–200. https://doi.org/10.2105/AJPH.2011.300608.
25. Major B, O'Brien LT. The social psychology of stigma. Annu Rev Psychol. 2005;56:393–421.
26. Mollborn S. Teenage mothers today: what we know and how it matters. Child Dev Perspect. 2017;11(1):63–9. https://doi.org/10.1111/cdep.12205.
27. National Women's Law Center. https://nwlc.org/resources/pregnancy-harassment-sexual-harassment-faqs-about-title-ix-and-pregnancy-harassment/
28. Noll JG, Shenk CE. Teen birth rates in sexually abused and neglected females. Pediatrics. 2013;131(4):e1181–7.
29. O'Keeffe GS, Clarke-Pearson K. The impact of social media on children, adolescents, and families. Pediatrics. 2011;127(4):800–4.
30. Osborne L. Beyond stigma theory: a literary approach. Issues Criminol. 1974;9(1, Spring):71–90.

31. Page R. Stigma. London: Psychology Press; 1984.
32. Saewyc EM, Magee LL, Pettingell SE. Teenage pregnancy and associated risk behaviors among sexually abused adolescents. Perspect Sex Reprod Health. 2004;36(3):98–105.
33. SmithBattle L. Reframing the risks and losses of teen mothering. MCN Am J Matern Child Nurs. 2009;34(2):122–8. https://doi.org/10.1097/01.NMC.0000347307.93079.7d. PMID: 19262267.
34. Seedat S, Scott KM, Angermeyer MC, Berglund P, Bromet EJ, Brugha TS, et al. Cross-national associations between gender and mental disorders in the world health organization world mental health surveys. Arch Gen Psychiatry. 2009;66(7):785–95. https://doi.org/10.1001/archgenpsychiatry.2009.36.
35. Thompson R. Sex in Middlesex: popular mores in a Massachusetts county, 1649–1699. Amherst: University of Massachusetts Press; 1986.
36. Turan JM, Elafros MA, Logie CH, Banik S, Turan B, Crockett KB, et al. Challenges and opportunities in examining and addressing intersectional stigma and health. BMC Med. 2019;17(1):7.
37. Vigod SN, Dennis CL, Kurdyak PS, Cairney J, Guttman A, Taylor VH. Fertility rate trends among adolescent girls with major mental illness: a population-based study. Pediatrics. 2014;133(3):e585–91.
38. Whitley R, Kirmayer LJ. Perceived stigmatisation of young mothers: an exploratory study of psychological and social experience. Soc Sci Med. 2008;66(2):339–48. https://doi.org/10.1016/j.socscimed.2007.09.014.
39. Wiemann CM, Rickert VI, Berenson AB, Volk RJ. Are pregnant adolescents stigmatized by pregnancy? J Adolesc Health. 2005;36(4):352.e8. S1054-139X(04)00456-2 [pii]
40. WHO Global health estimates. 2015: deaths by cause, age, sex, by country and by region, 2000–2015. Geneva: WHO; 2016.
41. Zeiders KH, Umaña-Taylor AJ, Jahromi LB, Updegraff KA, White RMB. Discrimination and acculturation stress: a longitudinal study of children's well-being from prenatal development to 5 years of age. J Dev Behav Pediatrics. 2016;37(7):557–64. https://doi.org/10.1097/DBP.0000000000000321.

The Intersection of Adolescent Development, Pregnancy, and Parenthood

4

Lois T. Flaherty and Sarah Lytle

Introduction

Both adolescence and parenthood are critical periods in the developmental cycle. Both involve profound changes in psychological functioning, and each can be seen as a developmental challenge or crisis.

Adolescence is a period of enormous change; it is the phase of life in which children become adults. Adolescence involves many developmental tasks—evolving a personal identity, renegotiating of relationships with parents, coming to terms with sexuality, and acquiring a capacity for intimacy, to name a few. In many ways, adolescents' physical abilities out-race their psychological ones. They sometimes take life-threatening risks before they learn to consider their consequences. They can bear children before they are ready to raise them.

Most individuals are able to navigate adolescence successfully to become independent adults capable of loving relationships and productive lives. However, there are many pitfalls in the trajectory from childhood to adulthood, as the individual is confronted with the physical changes of puberty and new social expectations. In addition, the brain undergoes significant transformation during adolescence and is not fully mature until adulthood. In the context of these significant social and psychological changes, adolescents are particularly vulnerable to stress.

In brief, adolescent development can be understood in the context of the individual's responses to biological imperatives and social expectations. The hormonal changes of adolescence are accompanied by a changing physical body, and new sexual feelings. As depicted in classical psychoanalytic theory, these biological changes propel the adolescent away from primary love objects, the parents, and

L. T. Flaherty (✉)
Harvard Medical School and Cambridge Health Alliance, Cambridge, MA, USA

S. Lytle
Case Western Reserve University, Cleveland, OH, USA
e-mail: sarah.lytle@uhhospitals.org

J.-V. P. Wittenberg et al. (eds.), *Adolescent Pregnancy and Parenting*,
https://doi.org/10.1007/978-3-031-42502-8_4

towards increasingly important relationships with peers and eventually, intimate partners. Attachment theory elaborated upon this shift, describing an evolution in the relationship with early attachment figures rather than a sundering of the bonds with them.

Social expectations of adolescents are culturally mediated and have varied over time. Historically, stages of life were conceptualized either as childhood or adulthood, with no intermediate state. Once children reached the age when they could become parents, they were expected to begin to take on adult roles. This is still true in some parts of the world, where early marriage and young parenthood are normative. In the industrialized world, there is an expectation that full adult functioning will not be reached until the mid-20s or later. In the USA and Canada and many other countries, a teen culture exists with a focus on peers, and particular styles of dress, hairstyles, and entertainment (fueled in affluent societies by the considerable purchasing power of adolescents and intense marketing to them). School becomes a pathway to college and future careers. Teenagers take on part time jobs and have the power to earn and spend money. They learn to drive. They engage in creative endeavors, such as sports, writing or art. In effect they are in a moratorium on taking adult responsibilities.

Adolescence has come to be conceptually divided into early, middle, and late periods, each with its own typical characteristics, although in actuality these developmental periods overlap and involve progressive and continual change and adaptation. Early adolescence is marked by the onset of menses in girls or first ejaculation in boys. This phase is characterized by increased affective instability, which in healthy adolescents progresses to the ability to manage affect and not be overwhelmed by it. As development proceeds, affect becomes increasingly differentiated, with a growing ability to express a range of emotions and to appreciate the feelings of others. Middle adolescence (ages 15–16) is usually the period of most conflict with parents as well as intensification of group identification. Initiation of sexual activity is common during this phase. Late adolescence (17–19) is characterized by a focus on identity and preparation for adult roles, which continues into what is now called emerging adulthood (20–25). Although adolescent pregnancy can occur at any time after menarche, it is most common during late adolescence; in 2019, 76% of all teen births occurred to 18–19-year-olds [34].

Pregnancy and Parenthood as a Developmental Crisis

Pregnancy at any age places new demands on the individual—a reconfiguration of identity, an orientation toward the future, and the acceptance of sharing one's body with another being. Teen pregnancy and motherhood, like other life challenges, call upon the individual to elaborate a new identity and perform a new social role, reconfiguring relationships with peers, parents, and of course with a child. She must call upon existing strengths, and also develop new resources for coping with the demands of motherhood. As with other crises, there is the potential for emotional growth and progression, as well as a danger of developmental arrest and regression.

Generally, the intrapersonal reorganization that accompanies pregnancy and parenthood have been considered as part of an adult developmental stage; hence most research has focused on adults. Psychoanalysts have been interested in the psychological aspects of pregnancy and motherhood from the early days, beginning with Freud's conceptualization of pregnancy and motherhood as the woman's compensation for not having a penis (See [8] for a systematic dismantling of that view). Since that time, as research and thinking have evolved beyond the limited perspective of Viennese patriarchal society, the psychology of pregnancy is understood as a complex process involving a redefinition of the self, with maternal feelings and a sense of oneself as a mother emerging out of the integration of intrapsychic and interpersonal experience [4].

With menarche comes the potential for pregnancy. The awareness of having a uterus and the potential to bear children is an important aspect of identity development. This awareness has been described as an awareness of "inner space" [14] and forms part of the woman's gender identity, self-concept, and body image. For most girls, menarche signifies the beginning of their trajectory towards adulthood, and the potential for pregnancy and childbearing. Later in adolescence a sense of oneself as a future parent begins to develop.

We know throughout history that for many women, pregnancy and childbirth have occurred soon after menarche. It is only in modern, technologically oriented societies that there is a long delay between the capacity to bear children and actual childbearing. For women in modern societies, an orientation toward the future (commonly referred to as "waiting"), is "incorporated into the female self-concept and becomes part of those characteristics of women that are developmentally related to her female body image" [38].

A new psychic reorganization occurs in response to the physical and psychological changes of pregnancy. Psychologically, both mothers and fathers begin to imagine themselves as parents, thinking about how they will care for the child. This has been described as activating a "caregiving system" [49], which will allow the parents to foster and take care of the child.

The development of a maternal identity is also part of this process of reorganization. The expectant mother's identity begins to incorporate a mental representation of the self as a mother, together with a mental representation of the future baby [1, 47].

Daniel Stern has described how maternal representations of the fetus evolve and increase in richness and specificity from the 4th to the 7th month of pregnancy, and then become less elaborate in the final trimester, only to be "re-elaborated" after the birth [50]. It is as if toward the end of her pregnancy the expectant mother begins to make space in her mind for the actual infant (in contrast to the fantasized infant). Postnatally, these representations can be distorted either positively or negatively—a child can be seen as wonderful and perfect (the best baby in the world) or as difficult and rejecting. Maternal representations are linked to the mother's own narrative about her experience of being mothered, which often undergoes a reworking during pregnancy. At the same time, a feeling of connection to the child and a sense of the child as a separate being develops—both important components of a maternal attachment system [1, 16, 29].

Pregnancy can be seen as a normal life crisis: that is, a phase in which an individual is confronted by new challenges and demands for adaptation. The key aspects of the developmental crisis of pregnancy are adjusting to the intrusion of the fetus, then the separation and loss of the fetus, and finally restoring the feeling that the body is whole [38]. Also necessary are anticipation and preparation for childbirth and motherhood, which may be accompanied by anxiety. There is a shift in attention from focusing on oneself and the relationships with significant others to the relationship with the unborn child.

For motherhood, the adaptive demands include: (1) functioning adequately in a maternal role, (2) feeling a sense of competence in doing so, and (3) being able to understand and respond sensitively to a child's emotional and physical needs. Societal expectations about the role are crucial, as are role models and social support.

The optimal outcome of this developmental crisis is a mastery of the role of the parent. To what extent this occurs will be influenced by many factors including the individual's level of maturity, social support, stress, and cultural factors. Grete Bibring pointed out over 60 years ago:

> What was once a crisis with carefully worked out traditional customs of giving support to the woman passing through this crisis period, has become at this time a crisis with no mechanisms within the society for helping the woman involved in this profound change of conflict solutions and adjustive tasks [4, p. 118].

While this is not necessarily true in all cases, as many women do have resources available to help them during this period, it is true that many modern societies tend to lack institutionalized mechanisms of support for pregnant women and new parents, and, certainly historically in the USA there has been a lack of support for pregnant and parenting adolescents.

The Adolescent Brain

Although there is much that remains to be understood, dramatic advances in neuroscience and studies of cognition have greatly increased our understanding of adolescent development. This knowledge has had a major impact on our understanding of adolescent behavior.

During adolescence, the brain undergoes growth and fine-tuning. There is growth in brain volume, especially in the frontal lobe. The prefrontal cortex (PFC), the last part of the brain to mature, progressively develops into early adulthood. The PFC is the brain's control center. It receives information from other parts of the brain, namely sensory and emotional information, processes it, and determines appropriate responses. Processing of information includes selectively attending to relevant stimuli and screening out or ignoring irrelevant stimuli. Although the prefrontal cortex is more mature in adolescents compared to children, it is not fully developed until early adulthood, or the mid-twenties [33]. This development, beginning around age 11, appears to involve both myelination of axons and, in the parietal and frontal areas, synaptic pruning, with the result that the gray areas are thinned, while the white matter volume increases. It is thought that synaptic pruning enhances connectivity among neurons and makes processing more efficient. In addition, there is believed to be (based on evidence from animal studies) an increase in dopaminergic activity and a "remodeling" of the dopaminergic system in conjunction with what has been termed the socio-emotional system (the amygdala, orbitofrontal cortex, insula, medial prefrontal cortex, and superior temporal cortex). This socio-emotional system, as well as other brain structures that involve emotional sensitivity and reward seeking, develop ahead of the PFC and are also influenced by hormonal changes of puberty [6].

Two important and overlapping features of cognitive functioning, executive functioning, and reflective functioning, are key to the successful completion of the developmental tasks. These functions are in turn the result of brain maturation. For them to develop optimally, social and environmental support is key.

Executive Functioning

Central to the control of behavior and emotion, executive functioning (EF) allows individuals to inhibit and modify their behavior to avoid undesirable consequences and thus maintain their pursuit of long-term goals. EF comprises abstract thinking, judging consequences of behavior, planning, and decision-making. Executive function includes the ability to manage time and attention, switch focus, plan and organize, remember details, curb inappropriate speech or behavior, and integrate past experience with present action. Two crucial components of EF are working memory, or the capacity to hold information on-line, and cognitive flexibility, or the ability to figure out how best to respond to new situations.

Both early childhood and early adolescence are peak periods for the development and maturation of EF [58]. EF varies considerably among individuals, and research suggests that patterns of executive functioning that are measurable in early childhood tend to persist into adulthood. Impairment in EF is typically found in attention-deficit disorder. Adverse childhood experiences also play a role, with adolescents with histories of childhood abuse showing impairment in EF, and the degree of impairment being proportional to the amount of abuse [36].

The Executive Functioning and Risk-Taking

An increase in risk-taking behavior is one of the hallmarks of adolescence [42]. Such behavior is normative and a necessary part of development, allowing for increasing independence and separation from parents as well as the development of an independent identity and intimate relationships outside the family. However, immature EF also predisposes adolescents to engage in risky activities, such as unprotected sex, as well as to act on impulse.

Risk-taking is not the same as impulsive behavior. An adolescent may make a carefully considered decision to begin using marijuana, for example, based on his own assessment of the risks and benefits involved. The decision about whether to engage in a particular behavior involves many factors, including the perception of risk, the attractiveness of the perceived rewards, social influences, and so on. An example might be a decision to forego going to a party in order to study for an exam. Such a decision involves consideration of the long-term consequences of behavior, the complexity of one's social role, and the ability to plan and strategize. It involves integration of cognitive and emotional functioning—however, much one might want to go to the party, the knowledge that it is likely to have a negative impact on examination performance is considered and weighed. An adolescent who perceives that she has little to gain by foregoing immediate pleasures will have a very different calculus. For the adolescent who has limited educational and employment prospects, and lives in a society where motherhood is valued, childbearing may be the best of the limited options available. Such an adolescent may make a deliberate decision to have a child.

Impulse control, on the other hand, involves attention, motor control, and future orientation. It includes the ability to inhibit or suppress responses to stimuli—to stop and think before acting. For example, a teenager might decide to ignore taunts, rather than to get involved in a fight. Such inhibition involves a cognitive appraisal of the stimulus as well as the weighing of the pros and cons of various responses. Both risk-taking and impulsivity have psychological, social, and neurobiological bases.

The neurobiology of adolescent brain development involves more than maturation of the prefrontal cortex. There is evidence that processing of emotion-laden stimuli (termed affective processing) differs markedly between adolescents and adults. This evidence suggests that teenagers rely more "primitive" brain structures and use different brain pathways for processing emotion-laden stimuli. It supports the hypothesis that spur of the moment decisions, which involve on the spot interpretation of the motives and affects of others, are different in adolescents. This evidence provides a possible explanation for the fact that adolescents are able to make reasoned decisions about their health and medical treatment (usually with the support and guidance of their families) but at the same time are liable to faulty judgment when it comes to situations in which they feel highly emotionally aroused, attacked or threatened, misperceive the degree of danger involved to themselves or others, or fail to appreciate the consequences of their actions.

Casey et al. [6] have presented a model based on different rates of maturation of the PFC and the limbic system that explains why adolescents, who are actually less impulsive than children, are more likely to engage in risky behavior. They posit that the prefrontal cortex develops in a linear fashion from childhood to adulthood, with steadily increasing cognitive control and emotional regulation, but that the limbic system undergoes a rapid maturation beginning in early adolescence. It is the limbic system that is involved in reward-related behavior, motivation, and emotional reactivity. They hypothesize that it is the imbalance between the two systems that results in poor decision-making as well as impulsive and sometimes risky behavior in highly emotionally charged situations. In their words, "in emotionally salient situations, the more mature limbic system will win over the prefrontal control system" (p. 117). They further suggest that this imbalance, which promotes risk-taking and reward seeking, and corresponds with the development of sexual maturity, plays an adaptive evolutionary role in propelling the movement of individuals away from their families of origin and towards mates outside their families.

It is intriguing that research on the functioning of the adolescent brain has confirmed the insights of psychoanalytic theory, which posited that hormonally based increased strength of sexual and aggressive drives that occurred with the onset of puberty resulted in an imbalance between the id (the seat of the drives) and the ego (the center of control) [59].

Factors Influencing Executive Functioning

There is considerable individual variation in EF among individuals of the same age. This has been found in clinical as well as brain imaging studies [25, 55]. Both early childhood adversity and later stressful experiences can impair EF.

The influence of early childhood adversity on brain development has been well documented [35]. Studies have shown exposure to stress impairs functioning of the prefrontal cortex (PFC) in humans as well as adult animal models, with acute stress causing a rapid and dramatic loss of prefrontal cognitive abilities and chronic stress causing changes in the architecture of prefrontal nerve cells [2].

As if this were not enough, there is evidence that vulnerability to stress rises from late childhood to late adolescence, with adolescents aged 15–17 showing the most pronounced responses to stress as measured by stress-induced cortisol levels [28, 51].

Finally, many psychiatric conditions are associated with impaired executive functioning. Numerous studies have shown that EF is also impaired in children and adolescents with post-traumatic symptoms [39], conduct disorder [15], ADHD [54], and substance abuse [9], all of which are associated with elevated rates of teen pregnancy.

We know that prior traumatic stress increases the impact of subsequent stress. In addition, the fact that adolescence per se may be a time of increased sensitivity to stress makes this period a particularly vulnerable time for all adolescents. Given that teen moms are likely to have experienced early and ongoing adversity, they are at considerable risk for being negatively affected by both acute and chronic stress, including the inevitable stress of pregnancy and parenthood, in addition to the not inevitable but nonetheless prevalent stress of being stigmatized.

The Importance of Executive Functioning in Parenting

Effective parenting involves recognizing and attending to children's needs and at the same time integrating these responses with environmental demands. These activities are components of EF. Aspects of EF that are involved in mothering include cognitive flexibility and working memory. Cognitive flexibility is the ability to adapt and improvise in order to meet new challenges. It involves juggling tasks, repeatedly and rapidly prioritizing, and figuring out new approaches when something doesn't work. Cognitive flexibility is a basic ingredient of successful parenting. A parent must be continually prioritizing tasks and responding to unforeseen situations. A mother will have to figure out when to stop what she is doing immediately to attend to her baby's needs and when to let him wait for a brief time. A mother who is engrossed in a telephone conversation with a friend and hears her baby crying has to decide between alternative responses—ignoring the baby, ending the call, or attempting to soothe the baby. As her child becomes a toddler, she has to decide how much freedom does she let him have, balancing risks against benefits.

Working memory is the ability to hold multiple bits of information in mind simultaneously and consider how best to respond. It allows parents to regulate their responses to challenging behavior and respond in a way that fosters healthy development in the child—in other words it facilitates thinking about various responses to infant behavior before responding. Impairment in working memory is associated with automatic responses, that is the parent's response is not thought out and might be associated with fixed assumptions or beliefs (giving a child who cries a bottle immediately rather than considering various possible reasons for the distress). Poorer working memory is associated with harsh and abusive parenting, which not only hampers a child's regulation of affect and behavior but also reinforces oppositional behavior [11].

In a study comparing teen and adult maternal responsiveness and executive functioning, researchers observed mother-infant interactions in their homes and administered neuropsychological tests to measure cognitive flexibility and working memory [7]. They found that poorer performance in cognitive flexibility in teen mothers was related to lower maternal sensitivity, although this association did not hold for the adults. For both teen and adult mothers, poorer cognitive flexibility was associated with decreased infant-directed vocalizations. (Working memory did not seem to be correlated with maternal–child interactions for the teens, although there was a relationship among the adults).

While working memory is a product of brain maturation, it is not fixed, and there is abundant evidence that it is negatively impacted by stress. Beckerman et al. [3] were able to show that experimentally manipulating stress levels affected working memory and parent-child interactions among women who were already experiencing high levels of stress, while having minimal effects on women who were not stressed. While their study involved adults, who presumably had completed their brain development, the kinds of stresses included those that are also common to teen mothers, such as partner-related and parenting stress.

In summary, the lack of fully developed executive function is a factor in adolescent risk-taking behavior, including unprotected sex, which carries a risk of unplanned pregnancy. Executive functioning also plays an important role in mothering. At higher risk for early childhood trauma, teenage mothers are particularly vulnerable to stressors of pregnancy and motherhood, and without adequate support, these stressors may further impair their EF and ultimately their ability to master the role of the mother.

Interventions to Improve Executive Functioning

There have been many attempts to demonstrate efficacy of interventions to improve EF. These have chiefly focused on preschool and school aged children as well as older adults. Results have been mixed, with real world interventions, such as martial arts or specially developed school programs showing more robust results than interventions such as computerized training. No interventions specifically designed to improve EF in teen parents have been studied systematically, although many interventions for this population do focus on helping young parents with things like money management and budgeting, job-seeking, and ensuring physically safe environment [56]. But given that stress has such an impact on EF intervention, interventions to reduce stress should be prioritized. Diamond and Ling, in an excellent review of interventions to promote EF, note the importance of reducing stress and addressing social needs to improve EF, citing studies demonstrating impairment in EF in depression, loneliness and social isolation, as well as in conditions associated with poor health, such as obesity [12].

Reflective Functioning

Reflective functioning (RF), or the capacity to envision mental states in oneself and others, is essential to healthy development and plays a crucial role in parenting. Reflective functioning (RF) undergoes rapid change and development during adolescence.

The term reflective functioning was introduced by Fonagy and colleagues in the 1990s [21]. It is tied to the concepts of mentalization (the act of thinking reflectively) and theory of mind (the ability to understand another's thoughts and feelings) and seen as a necessary component of attachment. Reflective function operates both inside and outside of conscious awareness; it evolves from the earliest relationships and depends on interaction with the minds of others; it is a vehicle for regulating affect. It can be measured with the Adult Attachment Interview (AAI; [24]), which includes a Reflective Function Scale, as well as other instruments.

Linking the concept of RF to the work of William James [30] on the components of "me" and "I" within the self, Fonagy and Target state:

> Reflective function is the developmental acquisition that permits the child to respond not only to other people's behavior, but to his *conception* of their beliefs, feelings, hopes, pretense, plans, and so on. Reflective function or mentalization enables children to *"read" people's minds* [20, p. 697].

Arising out of RF, affect mirroring is a way in which a parent uses "facial and vocal expression to represent to the child the feelings she assumes him to have in such a way as to reassure and calm rather than intensify his emotions" ([18], p. 8). In this way, the self of the child is socially constructed. For optimal development, the parent has to mirror the infant's emotions in a way that is soothing and calming

("Affect-regulative mirroring"), rather than echoing or magnifying the fear or anxiety or rage the infant feels. Neuroscience research has identified *mirror neurons*, that is, neurons that are responsible for one's sensations and emotions overlap with those recruited when one perceives another's sensations and emotions [23].

Failures of attunement—inaccurate or non-contingent mirroring—interfere with the infant's ability to organize internal emotional states. In such cases, the infant fails to develop their own capacity for mentalization. This can occur because parents are unable to handle the infant's negative affect because of their own difficulties with emotion regulation. In extreme cases, a parent might be overwhelmed with feelings of rage at an infant's fussiness. They may feel that the child hates them and is deliberately being difficult. This will interfere with the child's development of an ability to read others' emotional states.

Reflective Functioning in Adolescence

Although the development of RF has been relatively well studied in young children [19], it has received relatively little attention in adolescents (unlike executive functioning, which has been studied extensively). Nevertheless, it appears likely that RF does undergo important changes in adolescence, as adolescents develop a capacity for intimate relationships, which require an appreciation and awareness of others' minds. Bleiberg has discussed how adolescents can regress and "defensively retreat from reflective function in the context of specific internal and/or external cues, and activate rigid, non-reflective internal models built on the basis of discontinuities of experience and not integrated into the youngster's evolving autobiographical narrative" [5, p. 366].

Fonagy [17] has described the tremendous shift that must take place during adolescence if the young mother is to shift successfully from a primary attachment to her parents to herself becoming an object of attachment for her child. He sees the roots of many problems in adolescence as resulting from the teenager's being inadequately prepared to "reconfigure representations of relationships in line with the evolutionary and social demands of adolescence" [17, p. 334] by virtue of faulty attachment prior to adolescence. He links the antisocial and rebellious behavior of adolescence with oppositional-defiant behavior in young children, seeing both as manifestations of derangements in attachment, particularly the disorganized type of attachment, in which the child loves and cares for the parent, but also fears them.

Reflective Functioning and Parenting

Mothers and other caregivers are faced with interpreting their infants' behavior in the context of a non-verbal and rather limited behavioral repertoire for communicating wants and needs as well as emotional states. They are forced to rely on their own mental processes as well as whatever cues are forthcoming from the infant. For example, crying occurs for many reasons—hunger, pain, tiredness—and it is up to the baby's caretaker to interpret the meaning (as well as to understand that sometimes they have no idea why the baby is crying and not to feel guilty about this).

An appropriate maternal response depends on the mother's ability to accurately interpret the motivation underlying the child's behavior. At the same time, the baby's very limited behavioral repertoire makes this a difficult task, with the pitfall that the interpretation of the baby's signals may be primarily a projection of the mother's own thoughts and feelings. A mother who is insecure about her ability to care for her baby may feel the infant's crying as a criticism of her own ability to adequately care for her infant. She is likely to respond defensively, and in extreme cases may even respond punitively, seeing the behavior as willfully antagonistic. Or, as Schechter and Willheim have stated, "A caregiver in a state of defensive inhibition will be incapable of accurately responding to and reflecting the child's mental state, leaving the child to manage states of arousal and anxiety on their own" [45, p. 675].

The mother's ability to see the infant as a separate being with her own feelings and motivations arises out of her capacity for reflective functioning. One can see roots of this concept in the developmental theory of separation-individuation, where a failure of separation is associated with a fusion of the mental representation of the other with the self and with a variety of dysfunctional attachments outlined by Fonagy and colleagues (avoidant, dismissive and disorganized).

An important line of research has explored the relationship between maternal RF and infant development. As Fonagy and Target have emphasized, mother-child interaction plays a key role in the child's capacity for reflective functioning [19, 20]. Maternal RF has been shown to be important in the development of RF in the infant, and to facilitate secure attachment, cognitive development, and regulation of emotions and behavior [26]. It has been hypothesized that the mother continues to play a crucial role in helping the child develop RF in later years, by containing and transforming the child's experiences [31].

Reflective Functioning in Teen Parents

Young maternal age is a risk factor for low levels of RF [10]. In terms of RF, young mothers face particular challenges. For most teen parents, their child is their first, and like all new mothers, they face the problem of lack of experience. Second, their psychological development is incomplete, so their RF is not fully developed. At the same time parenthood provides an opportunity for further developing RF. By empathizing with their children, parents' reflective functioning is enhanced. Infants provide feedback to caregivers about the degree to which their communications are understood in the form of their behavior, and this behavior can be very reinforcing—for example, a baby's smile in response to her caregiver delights the caregiver; a baby whose distress is soothed by empathic caregiving rewards their caregiver by ceasing to cry.

The Impact of Stress on Reflective Functioning

While not specifically focused on adolescents, many studies have found low levels of parental RF in populations with histories of various types of childhood adversity, including abuse and neglect, substance abuse, family dysfunction, and parental psychopathology, as well as in minority and economically disadvantaged groups [10]. All of these studies suggest stress is a significant impedance to the development of RF.

One study that looked at RF in a group of pregnant teens from a socially disadvantaged population found generally low levels of RF, with participants varying in their ability to consider the future, reflect on their own experiences, and see their babies as separate individuals with their own needs [43].

Additional empirical evidence that stress can interfere with RF comes from the finding that mothers who have various psychiatric conditions have inaccurate perceptions about their infants. For example, mothers with depression or anxiety tend to report more behavior problems in their children [37]; conversely, non-depressed mothers compared to those with depression endorse less parenting stress, find their infants to be less difficult, and are more sensitive than depressed mothers [13]. Adolescents with more internalizing and externalizing behaviors of their own and lower levels of self-esteem are more likely to rate their infants as having more difficulties [46]. While psychiatric disorders are associated with impairment on many levels and the mother-child interaction is bidirectional, it is plausible that the misperception of the child 's behavior is mediated by impaired or incompletely developed RF.

In summary, RF is essential to healthy adolescent development, and parental RF is a crucial component of infant development. Much is unknown about adolescent RF and this is a crucial area for research in adolescence, but the evidence we do have suggests that the development of RF is hindered by psychosocial adversity, and much of teen pregnancy occurs in adverse social environments.

Interventions to Improve Reflective Functioning

Based on theoretical understanding of the role of RF in normal and pathological development, as well as observational studies of mother-infant interactions, interventions have been developed with the goal of enhancement of maternal RF. The basic idea is to teach parents to think about what the baby is thinking and feeling, rather than focusing on the behavior alone. Such interventions use techniques such as "speaking for the baby"—that is, interpreting the baby's behavior for the parent. For example, the therapist might point out how the baby follows his mother with his eyes and how this signifies how important she is to him, or how the baby's gestures and vocalizations indicate attempts to engage the parent. It may involve reframing of what the parent sees as negative behavior in a positive light.

Substance abusing parents, a group identified as deficient in RF [22, 52] and at very high risk for having children removed from their care, have been studied in terms of the impact of interventions to improve RF, with promising results [22, 32, 40, 41, 53]. Similar results have been found in mothers with prenatal depression [44].

Minding the Baby (MTB)® [48] is an evidence-based program to enhance reflective functioning in high risk first time young mothers aged 15–25 (60% are teens). In 2014 it was designated by the Health and Human Services Administration as one of 18 evidence-based home visiting programs in the USA.

The program, which serves a low-income urban population, involves weekly home visits by a nurse practitioner and social worker, who provide mother-infant therapy as well as case management services, beginning during pregnancy and continuing until the child is 2 years old. The therapy focuses on enhancing the mother's capacity to mentalize about her child's thoughts and feelings and to consider his behavior in light of his mental states. Results of a controlled study showed significant gains in RF among the mothers in the intervention group compared to a randomized control group who received routine prenatal and post-natal care. Equally impressive were the differences in attachment between the two groups, with the infants in the intervention group more likely to be securely attached and less likely to have disorganized attachments.

Baby Love is a 12-week program designed and developed by Dr. Jean Wittenberg at the Hospital for Sick Children in Toronto [57]. It is aimed at improving parents' understanding of their babies' thoughts, feelings, and perceptions, and improving their ability to cope with their emotional responses to the baby. Sessions are focused on topics such as:

What is Baby Feeling?

What is Baby Thinking?

Mindfulness in Parents and Understanding what Baby Perceives

Problem Solving

Parental Self-Regulation- Coping with Difficult Feelings and Thoughts Evoked by Baby

Coping with Anxiety

Coping with Feelings of Sadness and Depression

Parental Anger

Anger and Violence in the Family and in the Neighborhood

Selecting Alternate Caregivers

Summary

In summary, adolescent psychological development involves responding to the physical changes associated with evolution to adulthood, as well as increasingly complex cognitive, social, and emotional functioning. Pregnancy and parenthood likewise impose demands on the individual to think, feel, and act in new ways. In our previous report [27], we described teen pregnancy as interfering with normal adolescent development, essentially truncating it by depriving the adolescent of attending to her own developmental needs and forcing her to respond to a whole set of new demands and expectations more appropriate for adults. The fact that many teen pregnancies occur in already vulnerable young women makes the challenges they face even more daunting.

An understanding of adolescent development as well as the psychology of pregnancy and parenting can help to guide interventions to improve outcomes. It is especially important to recognize the noxious effects of stress on teen parents and their babies and to do everything possible to mitigate this. In addition, there are efficacious interventions to optimize parenting capacity. Pregnancy and the early years of infancy are critical times to intervene in promoting parental executive and reflective functioning. These interventions should be incorporated into programs for adolescent parents and parents-to-be, and studied systematically, so that the evidence base for promising interventions such as these that could help teen parents to become well-functioning adults and improve their ability to promote healthy development in their infants can be expanded.

References

1. Ammaniti M, Baumgartner E, Candelori C, Perucchini P, Pola M, Tambelli R, Zampino F. Representations and narratives during pregnancy. Infant Ment Health J. 1992;13:167–82.
2. Arnsten AFT. Stress weakens prefrontal networks: Molecular insults to higher cognition. Nat Neurosci. 2015;18(10):1376–85. https://doi.org/10.1038/nn.4087.
3. Beckerman M, van Berkel SR, Mesman J, Huffmeijer R, Alink L. Are negative parental attributions predicted by situational stress? From a theoretical assumption toward an experimental answer. Child Maltreat. 2020;25(3):352–62. https://doi.org/10.1177/1077559519879760.
4. Bibring GL. Some considerations of the psychological processes in pregnancy. Psychoanal Study Child. 1959;14:113–21.
5. Bleiberg E. Attachment, reflective function and the treatment of adolescents with severe personality disorder. In: Gutton IP, Godenne G, editors. Personality and conduct disorders in adolescence. Proceeedings of the International Society for Adolescent Psychiatry V International Congress. Paris: GEORGE Éditeur; 2001. p. 365–81.
6. Casey BJ, Jones RM, Hare TA. The adolescent brain. Ann N Y Acad Sci. 2008;1124:111–26. https://doi.org/10.1196/annals.1440.010.
7. Chico E, Gonzalez A, Ali N, Steiner M, Fleming AS. Executive function and mothering: challenges faced by teenage mothers. Dev Psychobiol. 2014;56(5):1027–35. https://doi.org/10.1002/dev.21185.
8. Chodorow N. The reproduction of mothering: Psychoanalysis and the sociology of gender. 2nd ed. Berkley: University of California Press; 1999.
9. Crunelle CL, Veltman DJ, Booij J, Emmerik-van Oortmerssen K, van den Brink W. Substrates of neuropsychological functioning in stimulant dependence: a review of functional neuroimaging research. Brain Behav. 2012;2(4):499–523. https://doi-org.ezp-prod1.hul.harvard.edu/10.1002/brb3.65
10. Cyr C, Euser E, Bakermans-Kranenburg M, van IJzendoorn, M. Attachment security and disorganization in maltreating and high-risk families: A series of meta-analyses. Dev Psychopathol. 2010;22:87–108.
11. Deater-Deckard K, Bell MA. Maternal executive function, heart rate, and EEG alpha reactivity interact in the prediction of harsh parenting. J Fam Psychol. 2017;31(1):41–50. https://doi.org/10.1037/fam0000286.
12. Diamond A, Ling DS. Conclusions about interventions, programs, and approaches for improving executive functions that appear justified and those that, despite much hype, do not. Dev Cogn Neurosci. 2016;18:34–48. https://doi.org/10.1016/j.dcn.2015.11.005.
13. Emery J, Paquette D, Bigras M. Factors predicting attachment patterns in infants of adolescent mothers. J Fam Stud. 2008;14(1):65–90. https://doi.org/10.5172/jfs.327.14.1.65.
14. Erikson EH. Childhood and society (1993-98578-000). New York: WW Norton & Co; 1964.
15. Fairchild G, Hawes DJ, Frick PJ, Copeland WE, Odgers CL, Franke B, Freitag CM, De Brito SA. Conduct disorder. Nat Rev Dis Primers. 2019;5(1):43. https://doi.org/10.1038/s41572-019-0095-y.
16. Fava Vizziello G, Antonioli ME, Cocci V, Invernizzi R. From pregnancy to motherhood: the structure of representative and narrative change. Infant Ment Health J. 1993;14(1):4–16.
17. Fonagy P. Attachment in infancy and the problem of conduct disorders in adolescence: The role of reflective function. In: Gutton P, Godenne G, editors. Personality and conduct

disorders in adolescence. Proceeedings of the International Society for Adolescent Psychiatry V International Congress. Paris: George Éditeur; 2001. p. 319–44.
18. Fonagy P. Affect regulation, mentalization and the development of the self. 2nd ed. London: Karnac; 2004.
19. Fonagy P, Target M. Playing with reality: I. Theory of mind and the normal development of psychic reality. Int J Psychoanal. 1996;77:217–33.
20. Fonagy P, Target M. Attachment and reflective function: their role in self-organization. Dev Psychol. 1997;9:679–700.
21. Fonagy P, Steele M, Moran G, Higgit A. The capacity for understanding mental states: the reflective self in parent and child and its significance for security of attachment. Infant Ment Health J. 1991;12:201–18.
22. Fonagy P, Steele M, Steele H, Leigh T, Kennedy R, Matton G, et al. Attachment, the reflective self, and borderline states. In: Goldberg S, Muir R, Kerr J, editors. Attachment theory; social, developmental, and clinical perspectives. Hillsdale: Analytic Press; 1995.
23. Gallese V, Keysers C, Rizzolatti G. A unifying view of the basis of social cognition. Trends Cogn Sci. 2004;8(9):396–403.
24. George C, Kaplan N, Main M. Attachment interview for adults. Berkeley: University of California; 1984/1985/1996. Unpublished manuscript.
25. Goldenberg D, Telzer EH, Lieberman MD, Fuligni AJ, Galván A. Greater response variability in adolescents is associated with increased white matter development. Soc Cogn Affect Neurosci. 2017;12(3):436–44.
26. Grienenberger J, Kelly K, Slade A. Maternal reflective functioning, mother-infant affective communication, and infant attachment: Exploring the link between mental states and observed caregiving behavior in the intergenerational transmission of attachment. Attach Hum Dev. 2005;7:299–311.
27. Group for the Advancement of Psychiatry, Committee on Adolescence. Crises of Adolescence. Teenage Pregnancy: Impact on Adolescent Development. New York: Brunner/Mazel; 1986.
28. Gunnar MR, Wewerka S, Frenn K, Long JD, Griggs C. Developmental changes in hypothalamus-pituitary-adrenal activity over the transition to adolescence: Normative changes and associations with puberty. Dev Psychopathol. 2009;21:69–85.
29. Ilicali ET, Fisek GO. Maternal representations during pregnancy and early motherhood. Infant Ment Health J. 2004;25:16–27.
30. James W. The Principles of Psychology. New York: H. Holt and Company; 1890.
31. Jemerin JM. Latency and the capacity to reflect on mental states. Psychoanalytic Study of the Child. 2004;59:211–39.
32. Jenkins C, Williams A. The mother-baby prenatal group: Nurturing reflective functioning in a methadone-maintenance clinic. Journal of Prenatal & Perinatal Psychology & Health. 2008;22:163–80.
33. Kolk, SM, Rakic, P. Development of prefrontal cortex. Neuropsychopharmacol. 2022;47(1): 41–57. https://doi.org/10.1038/s41386-021-01137-9.
34. Martin JA, Hamilton BE, Osterman MJK, Driscoll AK. Births: final data for 2019 (National Vital Statistics Reports Volume 70, Number 2). Centers for Disease Control and Prevention; 2021. https://www.cdc.gov/nchs/data/nvsr/nvsr70/nvsr70-02-508.pdf – PDF
35. McEwen BS. Brain on stress: how the social environment gets under the skin. Proc Natl Acad Sci. U. S. A. 2012;109(Suppl. 2):17180–85. https://doi.org/10.1073/pnas.1121254109.
36. Mothes L, Kristensen CH, Grassi-Oliveira R, Fonseca RP, de Lima Argimon II, Irigaray TQ. Childhood maltreatment and executive functions in adolescents. Child Adolesc Mental Health. 2015;20(1):56–62. https://doi.org/10.1111/camh.12068.
37. Najman JM, Williams GM, Nikles J, Spence S, Bor W, O'Callaghan M, Le Brocque R, Andersen MJ. Mothers' mental illness and child behavior problems: Cause-effect association or observation bias? J Am Acad Child Adolesc Psychiatry. 2000;39(5):592–602.
38. Notman MT. The female body and its meanings. Psychoanalytic Inquiry. 2003;23(4):572–91. https://doi.org/10.1080/07351692309349052.

39. Nyvold O, Nygaard E, Augusti E-M, Tamnes CK. Unity or diversity of executive functioning in children and adolescents with post-traumatic stress symptoms? A systematic review and meta-analysis. Child Neuropsychol. 2021; https://doi-org.ezp-prod1.hul.harvard.edu/10.1080/09297049.2021.1979950
40. Pajulo M, Pyykkönen N, Kalland M, Sinkkonen J, Helenius H, Punamäki RL, Suchman N. Substance-abusing mothers in residential treatment with their babies: importance of pre- and postnatal maternal reflective functioning. Infant Ment Health J. 2012;33:70–81.
41. Pajulo M, Suchman N, Kalland M, Mayes L. Enhancing the effectiveness of residential treatment for substance abusing pregnant and parenting women: focus on maternal reflective functioning and mother-child relationship. Infant Ment Health J. 2006;27:448–65.
42. Ponton LE. The romance of risk: Why teenagers do the things they do. 1st ed. Basic Books; 1997.
43. Sadler LS, Novick G, Meadows-Oliver M. "Having a baby changes everything" reflective functioning in pregnant adolescents. J Pediatr Nurs. 2016;31(3):e219–31. https://doi-org.ezp-prod1.hul.harvard.edu/10.1016/j.pedn.2015.11.011
44. Salo SJ, Flykt M, Mäkelä J, Biringen Z, Kalland M, Pajulo M, Punamäki RL. The effectiveness of nurture and play: a mentalisation-based parenting group intervention for prenatally depressed mothers. Prim Health Care Res Dev. 2019;20. https://doi-org.ezp-prod1.hul.harvard.edu/10.1017/S1463423619000914
45. Schechter DS, Willheim E. Disturbances of attachment and parental psychopathology in early childhood. Child Adolesc Psychiatr Clin N Am. 2009;18(3):665–86. https://doi-org.ezp-prod1.hul.harvard.edu/10.1016/j.chc.2009.03.001
46. Sieger K, Renk K. Pregnant and parenting adolescents: a study of ethnic identity, emotional and behavioral functioning, child characteristics, and social support. J Youth Adolesc. 2007;36(4):567–81. https://doi.org/10.1007/s10964-007-9182-6.
47. Slade A, Cohen LJ, Sadler LS, Miller M. The psychology and psychopathology of pregnancy. Reorganization and transformation. In: Zeanah CH, editor. Handbook of infant mental health: research and clinical applications. 3rd ed. New York: Guilford Press; 2009. p. 22–39.
48. Slade A, Sadler L, De Dios-Kenn C, Webb D, Currier-Ezepchick J, Mayes L. Minding the baby a reflective parenting program. Psychoanal Study Child. 2005;60:74–100. https://doi.org/10.1080/00797308.2005.11800747.
49. Solomon J, George C. Defining the caregiving system: toward a theory of caregiving. Infant Ment Health J. 1996;17:183–97.
50. Stern DN. Maternal representations: a clinical and subjective phenomenological view. Infant Ment Health J. 1991;12(3):174–86. https://doi.org/10.1002/1097-0355(199123)12:3<174::AID-IMHJ2280120305>3.0.CO;2-0.
51. Stroud LR, Foster E, Papandonatos GD, Handwerger K, Granger DA, Kivlighan KT, Niaura R. Stress response and the adolescent transition: performance versus peer rejection stressors. Dev Psychopathol. 2009;21(1):47–68. https://doi-org.ezp-prod1.hul.harvard.edu/10.1017/S0954579409000042
52. Suchman NE, DeCoste C, Leigh D, Borelli J. Reflective functioning in mothers with drug use disorders: implications for dyadic interactions with infants and toddlers. Attach Hum Dev. 2010;12:567–85.
53. Suchman N, DeCoste C, Castiglioni N, Legow N, Mayes L. The mothers and toddlers program: preliminary findings from an attachment-based parenting intervention for substance-abusing mothers. Psychoanal Psychol. 2008;25:499–517.
54. Toplak ME, Jain U, Tannock R. Executive and motivational processes in adolescents with Attention-Deficit-Hyperactivity Disorder (ADHD). Behav Brain Funct. 2005;1(1):1–8. https://doi.org/10.1186/1744-9081-1-8.
55. van Duijvenvoorde ACK, Huizenga HM, Somerville LH, Delgado MR, Powers A, Weeda WD, Casey BJ, Weber EU, Figner B. Neural correlates of expected risks and returns in risky choice across development. J Neurosci. 2015;35(4):1549–60. https://doi-org.ezp-prod1.hul.harvard.edu/10.1523/JNEUROSCI.1924-14.2015

56. Wittenberg J-V. Inventory for independent living for young mothers and babies. Toronto: Author; n.d.. Available from author at jean.wittenberg@sickkids.ca
57. St-André M, Reebye PN, Wittenberg JV. Infant mental health in Canada: initiatives from British Columbia, Québec and Ontario. J Can Acad Child Adolesc Psychiatry. 2010;19(2):116–23.
58. Zelazo P, Carlson S. Hot and cool executive function in childhood and adolescence: development and plasticity. Child Development Perspectives. 2012;6(4):354–60.
59. Freud, A. The ego and the mechanisms of defense (Rev. ed.). New York: International Universities Press; 1966.

Young Fathers

5

Jake Crookall

Introduction

Adolescent pregnancies are frequently impugned in media, politics, and public health. These discussions draw on associational data in a way that is congruent with societal stigma of adolescent pregnancy, such that, almost universally, adolescent pregnancy is deemed to "cause" a swath of adverse health consequences for the offspring. We have discussed the presence and harmful effects of this stigma towards adolescent mothers and children in other chapters of this book, however, I will turn now to discuss the fathers of these children. I argue that a similarly pernicious but distinct phenomenon occurs. Fathers' narratives are often also reduced to a problematic "single story"; a socially defined assumption of how these fathers' actions are responsible for their and their children's and the adolescent mother's poor health. Fathers in these families are often viewed as irresponsible and absent or at least uninterested in parenting. They are often depicted as antisocial personalities and generally assumed to be older males taking advantage of young, vulnerable females [15]. There can be many challenges associated with a "single story" of adolescent fathers which, intentionally or not, may reinforce power differentials that further poor health outcomes for these fathers and their families. Interventions exist that could benefit these fathers and their children; however, these are scarcely available and poorly studied due to institutional manifestations of this same stigma.

Poverty, racial, and ethnic minority status are associated with becoming an adolescent parent within the USA, however, these characteristics do not define all adolescent fathers. In stark contrast to this depiction are just a few celebrities who became fathers at a young age: rapper Lil Wayne became a father at age 15. Brian Jones, founder of the Rolling Stones, became a father at age 17. Levi Johnston, at

J. Crookall (✉)
Northern Ontario School of Medicine, Thunder Bay, ON, Canada

Lake of the Woods District Hospital, Kenora, ON, Canada

J.-V. P. Wittenberg et al. (eds.), *Adolescent Pregnancy and Parenting*,
https://doi.org/10.1007/978-3-031-42502-8_5

age 18, fathered a child with his fiancée, Sarah Palin's daughter, just months after Sarah Palin's failed vice-presidential bid in 2008. Basketball superstar LeBron James became a father at age 19 [25, 30]. These serve as some examples contrary to the typical vision conjured by the thought of adolescent fathers.

In an aim to complicate this "single story" of adolescent fathers further and to generate more inclusivity it is important to acknowledge that some families will not include a "mother" and "father" as are typically described in the literature. The current traditional description of parenting roles limits the range of discussion possible and may further marginalize sub-populations by failing to study or address their concerns. Some parents prefer non-gendered descriptions such as "parent." Some trans-male fathers will be the ones to carry and deliver a child. Same-sex couples may involve two fathers or none. Furthermore, atypical family relationships can result in multiple co-parents and in some cultures, especially with adolescent parents, caregiving may be done by grandparents or extended relatives, who themselves at times are known to the child as "mother" and "father." The assumptions and simplifications made by researchers in capturing and categorizing data often makes these populations invisible in the already limited literature that exists for adolescent parents. Furthermore, even with limiting the conversation to cisgender male parents in monogamous heterosexual relationships, there remains huge variability. More than their older counterparts, adolescent mothers are more likely to be in non-traditional parenting roles and are more likely to be single parents [15]. Over time, atypical family constellations have become the norm; the percentage of USA children living with two married parents in their first marriage has shrunk from 73% in 1960 to 46% in 2013 [18].

According to one nationally representative USA study, 10% of male respondents indicated a pregnancy before age 20. Of those fathers completing the in-depth interview associated with the National Longitudinal Adolescent to Adult Health study, nearly 80% (460 of the 597 sampled) reported their partners continued the pregnancy on to live births. As the authors note, abortions are typically under-reported and particularly so by males, suggesting the overall pregnancy rate for adolescent males in the USA may be even higher [10]. This study, titled "Male abortion beneficiaries…" goes on to outline associational data that those fathers who reported their partner had an abortion described higher educational attainment although not higher economic attainment; a striking outcome given that the study likely contained residual confounding in that adolescents from higher-income families would be more likely to have partners who chose abortion. From the author's choice of the title of the article, their opinion that adolescent fathers should benefit from the pregnancies being aborted is clear, despite this contrasting with one of the studies main findings. This article serves as a microcosm of challenges facing approximately 8% of American fathers—that despite evidence that fails to support the hypothesis, the scientific community conveys that adolescent fatherhood is a cause of negative outcomes.

Fatherhood is a culturally defined construct and thus expectations of a father vary widely with individuals' cultural and personal history. Expectations may range from an anticipation the father will never meet their child to expecting him to be the primary caregiver. Across the USA and reflected in much of the academic literature on parenting is an expectation that the father's role with the family is more instrumental—to support the mother financially and perhaps emotionally. These biases are implemented in our institutions. A qualitative analysis of 25 African American adolescent fathers who were actively engaged in prenatal care highlights some of the challenges: prenatal appointments scheduled during the day often conflict with work and school schedules; neutralizing reactions by health care practitioners, such as leaving a father in the waiting room or not speaking with him during clinical encounters; and distancing reactions such as a nurse stating to a father in the study after he enthusiastically voiced pride at the birth of his child *"How many babies does this make?"* embarrassing the young couple by implying the young man had fathered many children [7]. These acts of prejudice by health care providers and others may cause fathers to feel less confidence in their role as fathers and thereby participate in them less.

Part of the challenges to supporting young fathers during this time includes the frequent age, racial and socio-economic differences between the demographic becoming adolescent parents and the demographic of those providing care and completing research on this group, which authors highlight as one potential origin for some of these differences in the expected role of adolescent fathers [7]. A number of those few resources that do exist have taken root within the context of programs founded to support adolescent mothers. Research in the field has often depended upon mother's report of the father's behavior rather than interacting directly with the fathers as studies often capture participants from their prenatal appointments. As such, the perspective of adolescent fathers is rarely included in clinical and policy decision-making. Of note, in the production of this book we have included the perspective of an adolescent mother throughout the writing process, however we have not been able to engage an adolescent father in the review of this chapter, let alone the writing process of the book from the outset, as would be preferable.

Legislation regarding child support payments largely assumes that fathers are already at a place where they are obtaining an income and has limited allowance for fathers who may still be completing secondary or post-secondary schooling as outlined by Kiselica [18]. Legislation around access typically provides for an assumption that the mother is the custodial parent, unless otherwise determined—reflecting a culturally sanctioned underlying assumption, at least historically, that the mother's interactions with the child are of greater importance than those of the father. These assumptions about fathers—particularly that their primary role in raising a child is their financial contribution—can be particularly problematic with adolescent fathers and contribute towards their lack of involvement with their children. Adolescent fathers, who may have not yet completed high school, may drop out to gain immediately available and often low-paying work to provide for their children. Others may avoid claiming paternity, to avoid mandatory child support payments, but also thereby forfeit rights to access and emotionally support their child. A system designed around the role of the father as a social support would encourage these fathers to remain in contact with their child. Financial policies that supported paternity could increase the number claiming paternity, and by strengthening bonds between the father and child would likely increase the long-term social-emotional, instrumental, and financial support provided across the child's lifespan. Policies that provide sufficient universal funding for families or targeted supports to fathers could also encourage fathers to continue their own development, potentially upgrading their education and thereby have more to provide for their families. Some advancements have been made along this course, including the Federal Fatherhood Initiative undertaken by then President Bill Clinton, and George W. Bush's further support. Funding was provided to target increasing father involvement, as 60% of children born in the 1990s would spend a significant portion of their childhoods without a father in the home, with associations to poverty and antisocial behavior. One program that highlighted the involvement of fathers was the Parents' Fair Share program which involved employment, training services, peer support groups, voluntary mediation between parents, and modified child support enforcement. It led to increased employment, income, active parenting, and more child support payments [15].

Within healthcare and academia, these biases against involvement of adolescent fathers are also reflected. Most of the research completed with young families is done through programs in place to support adolescent mothers. They are often extensions of research geared to understand women's experience and may rely on mothers' reports of the fathers' experiences. Clinical programs for young mothers understandably have a focus to create safe environments for these women; however, in doing this often exclude fathers altogether, even in the cases where the relationship is supportive, and the father is seeking to be engaged in the family. This might be done in overt or more subtle, structural means. For example, a clinic which sees the mother as the patient may not have capacity to see the father as a patient, and may not involve the father in parenting strategies given he, nor the child, are the identified patient. Without a parallel program geared towards fathers, or one that adopts a combined approach with a mandate to treat all members of the family; these fathers are left without care and receive a message that they are not integral to key elements of their child's life, such as their medical appointments. These messages may then be internalized, and the father may stop making efforts to be included in these and other aspects of the child's life.

Challenges inherent to studying adolescent fathers includes their lower prevalence than teen mothers, issues of uncertain paternity in epidemiologic studies, and greater inaccuracies in reporting of age in younger parents [23, 32]. Women under 18 may be concerned to give the identity or age of a sexual partner accurately, given potential charges of statutory rape that their partner could incur. Fathers may avoid claiming paternity due to concerns about having to pay child support, or retaliation from the mother's family [15].

Through this chapter, I will attempt to summarize evidence we have from fathering studies in general and the few studies we have of young fathers in particular. In providing these summaries, however, I ask that the reader keeps in mind the risks of these reductionistic statistics: that they do not necessarily reflect causality and certainly are not universally true for any particular young father they may encounter. Given the limited data and challenges with selection bias in the existing studies, the ability to generalize from many of these studies to a particular clinical encounter may also be a challenge. My goal by defining the mean experiences of this group is to provide readers with some information about this population, while avoiding the creation of a "single story" of adolescent parenting.

Describing Young Fathers in America

As described previously, the USA has more teen parents than any other developed country despite a significant recent decrease. The fertility rate decreased between 1991 and 2015 from 24.7 to 10.4 live births per thousand males aged 15–19 [23]. These shifting rates may also reflect a shifting demographic of who becomes an adolescent father, leaving some of the limited research reviewed above of questionable applicability to current young fathers. Despite these limitations, it is important for a clinician to be informed regarding these associations such that they can be screened for and addressed as clinically indicated. Individual factors including academic failure, aggressive behaviors, antisocial behavior; interpersonal associations including low popularity, "deviant" peer association and parental antisocial behavior; additionally, social factors such as family poverty have been associated with becoming a teen father [32]. Young fathers are less likely to be married to the mother of their children and less likely to cohabitate.

When discussing "young fathers" there are multiple groups one could consider, with different studies using different criterion to describe these fathers, including defining them as: male parents aged 15–19 [23]; male parents 24 years old or younger, to children with mothers aged 14–18 [13]; or as fathers less than 25 years old to children of women under 20 [11]. It is more common for fathers to be peers or older than the mothers; using California birth certificate data from 1993 Males and Chew [21] demonstrated that for a 17-year-old woman giving birth, approximately 20–28% of fathers would have been peers (age 17–18 years) whereas 47–50% would have been older youth (between 19 and 22 years), approximately a quarter (between 20% and 26%) being age 23 or older with only 4–5% of fathers expected to be younger teenagers (ages 15–16 years). One retrospective chart review noted that for very young mothers (<15 years) in California, 27% of births were to an adult male who was on average 8.8 years older. Notably in the research definitions for young fathers given above, none appear to capture the group of adolescent fathers who would have female partners over age 20, which thus would fail to capture a particular sub-population of adolescent fathers. This oversight likely reflects an institutional tendency to see adolescent fathers as accessory to the mother-infant dyad.

The age of the father appears to correlate with choices the mother makes around continuing her pregnancy. Unmarried pregnant women under 18 have lower rates of abortion with increasing ages of their partners: 61% of women who were in a relationship with a male who was also under 18 reported obtaining an abortion, compared to 57% for women with partners aged 18–19 years and 33% of women with male partners over 19 years [16]. One could speculate if this association may be related to expected financial stability with an older partner, potential differences in the male's wishes or the nature of the relationship that led a woman to decide to keep the pregnancy after becoming pregnant. It may also be that women who are seeking to have a child are more likely to choose older male partners. In attempting to guess at underlying causal associations in the context of limited data it is important to be aware of how our personal biases of this population may influence our assumptions and attributions of causality.

Factors associated with becoming an adolescent father appear to be maternal education, paternal education, number of children in the home of origin, single-parent homes, living with the biological father, having oneself an adolescent mother, having oneself an adolescent father, having "deviant" peers, dating early, substance use, race, and environments characterized to lack enrichment or be full of physical risk. Interestingly, when Sipsma et al. [29] conducted a fully-adjusted model, which takes into account other variables that might themselves explain some of these associations, adolescent motherhood was no longer a statistically significant independent variable in their cox regression model, whereas adolescent fatherhood remained significant; leading the authors to conclude that targeting adolescent fatherhood may be a means to prevent a second generation of adolescent fathers [29]. While it is concerning that the goal of this article appears to be solely reducing adolescent pregnancies, rather than addressing factors which might lead to hardship associated with the pregnancies, it does highlight the importance of including adolescent fathers in approaching care and policies with these marginalized and vulnerable populations.

Regarding the relationship pattern, it appears overall that adolescent compared to older mothers are less likely to be married or to cohabitate with the fathers of their children, although are desiring to become pregnant in most cases and hopeful to continue a romantic relationship with the father. One study of a sample of 18- and 19-year-old mothers in Genesee County, Michigan, observed the following: 21% of the women they studied became pregnant. At the time of becoming pregnant, 16% reported being married to their partner, 23% engaged, 21% cohabitating, and 17% were seriously dating. Twenty-seven percent of pregnant mothers indicated their partner had sex with another person, 75% described intimate partner violence. Compared to non-pregnant peers there was more than double the level of reported disrespect, more than triple the rate of physical threats and four times the rate of physical assault (21% of pregnant mothers); all these rates were significantly different than their non-pregnant peers. At the termination of the study, 39% of the relationships that lead to pregnancy broke up, a further 21% broke up at some point but got back together and 40% of the relationships were ongoing. This is significantly different from non-pregnant peers who were more likely to break up (76%) and less likely to break up then reunite (5%). After pregnancy, 22% of relationships became more serious, while 42% became less serious or broke up [2]. Additionally, the authors note there were likely further dissolution of relationships after the relatively short follow-up period of two-and-a-half years. This is significant as the partner's presence in the home and involvement in the family, have been strongly associated with child outcomes as will be discussed in the next section.

As family develops, it appears that the presence of a father in the home continues to be associated with other outcomes. Repeated pregnancy within 2 years is known to be more common among adolescent mothers. It has been a focus of health care interventions, given that the second child compared to second children born after more than 2 years delay, has been noticed to have higher rates of preterm births, mental health issues, and developmental problems. A variety of factors have been associated with a woman's reduced likelihood for a repeat pregnancy, including access to birth control, staying in school, and having good mental health. It was also noted that adolescent women who had a greater age difference with their partner, were cohabiting with a partner and who found their partner as supportive had more frequent repeat pregnancies. Noticeably, marital status was not associated with frequency of repeated pregnancy [22].

Young Father Involvement

Having outlined some of the characteristics of young fathers above, one challenge to highlight is the multiple barriers to father involvement for adolescent fathers. Father involvement has been defined as the level of engagement a father has with his child and with the mother of the child. It has increasingly been recognized as a determinant of outcomes for children and families. Different aspects of father involvement have been theorized to support child development; from instrumental support and emotional support to the mother, to direct interactions with the child [27]. Interestingly, comparing father's parenting across age, involvement tends to increase with older fathers, with teen fathers being the least engaged; although among all fathers who are not cohabiting with the child's mother, teens are the most likely to be engaged [4].

Some early psychodynamic theories of father involvement focused on the father's role of protecting the mother and infant from the outside world: "they not only felt themselves the feelings of their women, and went through some of the agony, but also they took part, warding off external and unpredictable impingements, and enabling the mother to become preoccupied, to have but one concern, the care of the baby that is there in her body or in her arms" [31]. Winnicott highlights the importance of the parental relationship to protect the infant by forming a "rock to which he can cling and against which he can kick" ([36], p. 115). Mahler and Gosliner [19] go on to identify the father as the child's initial contact outside of the mother-infant dyad and the agent responsible for promoting the child's understanding of themselves as separate from their relationship with their mother and to support their engagement with the outside word, in contrast to the mother's role of promoting self-discovery and self-regulation in the infant. In their words, ″The father … is a powerful and perhaps necessary support against the threat of re-engulfment of the ego into the whirlpool of the primary undifferentiated symbiotic stage″ [19, pp. 209, 210]. The intrusion of the father upon the mother-infant dyad is formulated at times as a helpful rescuer [13, 20] and sometimes as disruptive; on some occasions viewed as causing distress and fear in the child as the original "stranger" [8, 17].

Attachment theory, even as originally formulated by Bowlby [3], stipulates that the father provides another alternative attachment figure, noting that having a secure relationship with either parent was highly protective, beyond simply the security of the relationship with the mother. This would support the role of the father being more interchangeable with the role of the mother with regard to the child's ability to develop self-regulation, rather than distinct based on gender. More recent research has included a focus on triadic or broader family interaction cycles and how these family systems affect infant development. These patterns are highlighted in the work by Fivaz-Depeursinge and Philipp [11]. They note family relationships where parents are excluding, competing, or only connecting through their child and the impacts this can have on the child.

I suspect the variety in the psychodynamic theories regard the role of fathers in the family is itself a product of the many varying roles that fathers can have. In some cases, abusive or intrusive fathers likely have a highly disruptive role; in the case of absent or impaired mothering roles the father can likely function as a protective attachment figure and in triadic parenting relationships the father may also have roles of providing instrumental and emotional support to the mother's parenting role. In most cases the same father likely takes on these different roles fluidly at different times and the infant's view of the father thus is shaped with some of that complexity and based on the reactions of the mother towards the father as outlined in triadic theory. Different cultural views of the role of the father may shape how any individual father feels free to engage with their infant and thus their opportunity to serve as a valuable resource to this developing family. In the context of stigma associated with adolescent parenting, the concern is that adolescent fathers will be pushed towards roles of being only instrumentally supportive, or if not accepted by mothers and maternal extended families, adolescent fathers may be expected only to function as a disruption to the mother-infant bond, rather than being supportive to it and developing their own attachment relationship with the child.

As a backdrop for discussing the adolescent-specific literature, let us review some of the trends and findings that have been observed with fathers generally. Fathers have been identified to have impacts on their children directly and in the context of the relationship they have with the child's mother. Additionally, it has been demonstrated that healthy father involvement may mitigate some of the health and behavioral challenges observed among children of depressed mothers [5]. Father involvement, variably defined, has been associated with improved educational and health outcomes in their children and so is receiving increased attention. When studied on population levels, researchers have used whether a father's name is indicated on the birth certificate as a measure of father involvement; this measure of father involvement has been associated with lower perinatal mortality, with an adjusted relative risk estimated to be 80% greater for those who did not have a father listed.

Paternal involvement, as measured by father's name on birth certificate, has been associated with lower perinatal mortality in two studies, with adjusting for marital status [adjusted RR = 1.8 (1.6,2.0)] [1]. In pregnancies to teenage mothers, father's name on birth certificate was associated with decreased incidence of a variety of birth outcomes in adjusted analyses [adjusted OR 1.15 (1.12–1.18)]. Cost effectiveness modeling on a large retrospective trial indicated costs for father uninvolved pregnancies based on hospital admission costs in the first year of life, irrespective of parental age, to be between $1139 and $1827 [26].

In some communities, and arguably most commonly those with adolescent fathers, a "father deficit model" exists. This model views the father as ineffective or neglectful in supporting child health and development [16, 27] and can itself impede their involvement. Panter-Brick et al. [30] argue that fathers should be seen as co-parents whose involvement can be highly supportive of a child's development.

A 10-year longitudinal follow-up study by Howard et al. [14] of 134 adolescent mothers outlines the elements of father involvement based on the mother's report. The sample was predominantly of African American mothers and of individuals with low socio-economic status, originally recruited in the 1990s. Eight percent of the adolescent mothers reported being married prior to the birth of their child, which then increased to 20% of mothers by the time the child was 8 years old. The vast majority (90%) reported being in contact with the child's father just prior to delivery, whereas approximately two thirds (59%) of mothers reported ongoing contact with the father when the child was 8 years old. They reported the fathers of their children were on average 19 years old at the time of birth, and predominantly African American (68%), with 26% European American. Half of the children's fathers were reported to have graduated from high school by the time the child was age 6, with 9% having obtained further education and 67% being employed. Of women giving birth to a second child within 6 years of the birth of their first child, 34% had the same father [14]. Given this data is from one relatively small cohort which was collected over two decades ago, generalizing from these data to current adolescent fathers may be problematic, particularly given there have been significant shifts in the birth rate for adolescent mothers over this time as described above. It is interesting to note the significant drop-off of father involvement over the course of the child's life and to potential opportunity to intervene in a fashion that would increase fathers' ongoing involvement with their children where appropriate.

Kiselica [18] argues this pattern of father involvement both challenges the common narrative that teen fathers are antisocial members of society who abuse and force women to become pregnant without any interest in fathering; and suggests that existing stigma may create barriers that impair young father's ability to remain involved with their children, especially following a change in relationship status with the mother of their child. He suggests that navigating the double challenge of adolescent development and becoming a parent, in the context of often unsupportive families and health care systems, leads fathers to have increased tension in the relationship with their partners. He also suggests their lack of education regarding the importance of father involvement, an internalized social expectation of being uninvolved, personal histories of insufficient fathering, and a lack of knowledge regarding legal rights to access their child all serve as potential causal mechanisms for the decreased rates of young fathers' involvement, affecting over 175,000 males aged 15–19 per year in the USA alone. This opinion is supported by a study completed by Gavin et al. [12] which obtained information from 181 mothers under 20 years about the fathers of their children and discovered that the parental relationship status was the factor most strongly associated with father involvement.

Greater numbers of studies have been published in the adult literature allowing for some meta-analysis of their effectiveness, as reviewed by Sarkadi et al. [27] in a systematic review of 24 papers covering 16 different longitudinal studies of father involvement. Father involvement is defined variably, from cohabitation to engagement. They highlight only 18 of the studies controlled for SES in their analysis in any fashion. Of those 18, five described general positive effects of father involvement on offspring outcomes. Eleven described positive effects for certain subgroups, including those with poor families, adolescents with high-delinquency rates or African Americans. Behavioral, social, cognitive, and psychological effects were identified. These included improvements in rates of behavioral problems, educational outcomes, and functioning across childhood and adulthood. In poor families, stable marriages predicted lower incidence of criminality in offspring during adult years. Father involvement was associated with decreased homelessness or state benefits in adult life. At 3 years of age socially disadvantaged African American children had significantly higher IQ associated with daily father involvement, contrastingly in the National Survey of Children from the USA it was only socially advantaged populations that demonstrated improved educational attainment with father involvement. Of note, one of the papers included in the study did find negative effects (father involvement at age 6 was associated with increased hyperactivity at age 14) and another found no benefit of father cohabitation during the first 3 years on cognitive development. While there appears to be some variability, perhaps due to study design or populations sampled, the overall picture is that increased father involvement is repeatedly associated to significant improvements for their children across their lifespan.

Challenges with Research Methodology

Descriptions of adolescent fathers often highlight a variety of negative health outcomes associated with becoming a father at an early age, and quickly move to indicate adolescent parenting as a risk factor that should be prevented through sexual education and increasing access to birth control and abortion services. While these steps appear to reduce rates of adolescents' becoming fathers, the approach often pathologizes the state of being an adolescent parent to the detriment of those who are adolescent fathers. Discussion about the determinants of health that might lead to becoming an adolescent father and be responsible for the associated negative health outcomes appears absent in many of these discussions. Similarly, resources need to be directed to support those males who become parents as adolescents, as opposed to only placing resources into prevention. Of note, the associational data often cited to validate these claims is not sufficient to establish a causal relationship as the studies often fail to provide longitudinal follow-up in addition to failing to account for several potential confounders. A well-designed observational study on this topic would require longitudinal follow-up and measurement of basic

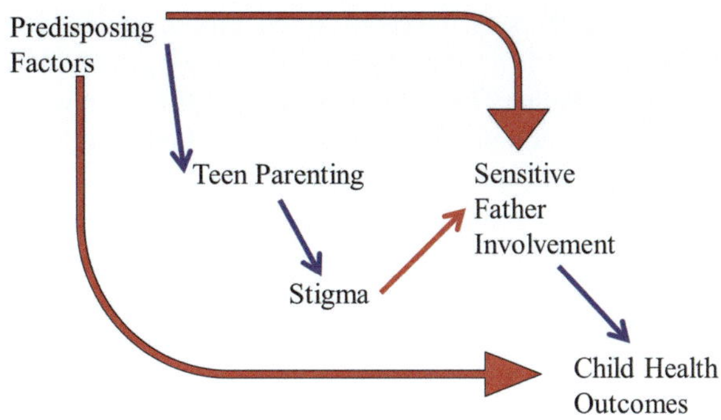

Fig. 5.1 Theorized DAG

demographic factors, details of the parents' history of traumatic experiences and relationship histories; environmental impacts, such as family and cultural beliefs about the adolescent father's involvement, which may impair his ability to access the child like how they would as an older father.

The theorized relationships between these variables are described in the Theorized Directed Acyclic Graph (DAG) below (Fig. 5.1), a tool in research to reduce potential bias [28]. Individual factors, including academic failure, aggressive behaviors, antisocial behavior; interpersonal associations including low popularity, deviant peer association and parental antisocial behavior; combined with social factors such as family poverty have all been associated with becoming a teen father [32].

In political discourses through much of the global north, teenage pregnancy and parenting has often been described as a "catastrophe" or "crisis" and dominant discourse often portrays teenage parents as "both a social threat and social victims" [9]. This is also true in healthcare, where medical homes have been created to support teen parents, although those involved while well-meaning may continue a number of harmful stereotypes. This is particularly visible in the frequent lack of engagement with adolescent fathers in such programs, despite evidence that between two thirds and three quarters of fathers are in a relationship with the mother at the time of giving birth [6], and that many of these couples have decided together to become pregnant. Rather than perpetuating the stigma that adolescent fathers are not active members of their family, our institutions can take an active role in reaching out and supporting their involvement.

Programs for Teen Fathers

The impact that adolescent fatherhood has largely been overshadowed by attention and emphasis placed on adolescent motherhood. There have been some programs developed to support teen fathers, following the explosion of adolescent mother programs in the USA as outlined by Kiselica [18]. In 1983 an eight-center collaboration, the Teen Father Collaboration was formed. An other notable program supporting adolescent fathers is a school-based group, the Maximizing A Life Experience. A third example is the multi-centre inter-agency coordinated effort called the Maine Young Fathers Project. Carl Mazza [24] demonstrated superiority in a comprehensive multi-component intervention including individual and group counseling, educational and vocational support, medical care, housing support, legal advocacy, recreational activities, and parenting skills training over parenting skills training alone. In Buffalo, New York, impoverished new and expecting adolescent fathers were given educational, employment and psychosocial support through the Fathers Forever Program. The Texas Fragile Families Initiative ran in eleven communities across the state offered comprehensive services in a mix of school and community- based locations. Unfortunately, this is the extent of programs geared to adolescent males identified in an intensive literature search, demonstrating limited academic work done documenting their impacts or cost effectiveness.

Conclusion

Adolescent fathers are common; estimates range up to 10% of American men father pregnancies before age 20. It appears that those who become adolescent fathers are more likely to be impoverished, have lower levels of education and have peers engaged in deviant behaviors and parents engaged in antisocial behaviors. Father involvement generally offers protective factors to offspring across their lifespan, and some limited evidence supports this association among adolescent parents as well. Despite this evidence, very few programs exist and even less evidence regarding their implementation to guide efforts. Instead, we have an academic environment that focuses on treating adolescent fathers as outcasts and adolescent fatherhood as a condition to be prevented through targeted public health interventions. Such interventions fail to address the socio-economic and social conditions impacting these fathers and their families. Additionally, societal pressures often block access for these fathers from their children, both preventing their rights to parent and their offspring's potential to benefit. Certainly, as with older fathers, there are some cases where partner abuse may limit their ability to be involved with the family; however, we cannot let our stigma of adolescent fathers as abusers contaminate our entire approach to supporting this vulnerable population. Indeed, for adolescent parents are often particularly primed to take advantage of resources available to them if offered at such a pivotal moment in a young man's life such as the birth of his child.

Informing young fathers of their importance to their child's development is likely a first approach to combat the stigma and existent societal pressures keeping them from parenting. Providing them with knowledge of their legal rights to access and custody of their children could increase father involvement beyond a point of dissolution of a relationship with the child's mother. Involving young fathers in the perinatal care of the baby would highlight the importance of this role and allow an opportunity for involvement of social supports where indicated. Addressing determinants of health and mental health concerns may help to reduce potential adverse outcomes such as the increased rates of intimate partner violence among adolescent fathers. Further study of these interventions is undoubtedly required; however, we already have evidence that robust multi-systemic interventions can improve outcomes for adolescent fathers and their children. Rather than concentrating efforts on reducing the phenomenon of adolescent parenting, robust investments in adolescent fathers have the potential to support already marginalized populations and generate significant and intergenerational returns on investment.

References

1. Alio, et al. Feto-infant health and survival: does paternal involvement matter? Matern Child Health J. 2010;14:931–7.
2. Barber JS, Kusunoki Y, Gatny H, Melendez R. The relationship context of young pregnancies. Law Inequal. 2017;35(2):175.
3. Bowlby J. A secure base: parent-child attachment and healthy human development. New York: Basic Books; 1988.
4. Castillo, Sarver. Nonresidential fathers' social networks: the relationship between social support and father involvement. Pers Relationsh. 2012;19:759–74.
5. Chang JJ, Halpern CT, Kaufman JS. Maternal depressive symptoms, father's involvement, and the trajectories of child problem behaviors in a US national sample. Arch Pediatrics Adoles Med. 2007;161(7):697–703. https://doi.org/10.1001/archpedi.161.7.697.
6. Clayton. The lives of young fathers: a review of selected evidence. Soc Policy Soc. 2016;15(1):129–40.
7. Dallas CM. Interactions between adolescent fathers and health care professionals during pregnancy, labor, and early postpartum. J Obstet Gynecol Neonat Nurs. 2009;38(3):290–9. https://doi.org/10.1111/j.1552-6909.2009.01022.x.
8. Diatkine R. Agressivité et fantasmes d'agression. Rev Franç Psychanal. 1966;30:15–92.
9. Duncan. What's the problem with teenage parents? And what's the problem with policy? Crit Soc Policy. 2007;27(3):307–34.
10. Everett BG, Myers K, Sanders JN, Turok DK. Male abortion beneficiaries: exploring the long-term educational and economic associations of abortion among men who report teen pregnancy. J Adolesc Health Off Publ Soc Adolesc Med. 2019;65(4):520–6. https://doi.org/10.1016/j.jadohealth.2019.05.001.
11. Fagan J. Randomized study of a prebirth coparenting intervention with adolescent and young fathers. Family Relations: An Interdisciplinary Journal of Applied Family Studies. 2008;57(3):309–23. https://doi.org/10.1111/j.1741-3729.2008.00502.x.
12. Fivaz-Depeursinge E, Philipp D. The baby and the couple: understanding and treating young families. London: Routledge; 2014. https://doi.org/10.4324/9781315779775.
13. Florsheim P, Burrow-Sánchez JJ, Minami T, McArthur L, Heavin S, Hudak C. Young parenthood program: supporting positive paternal engagement through coparenting counseling. Am J Public Health. 2012;102(10):1886–92. https://doi.org/10.2105/AJPH.2012.300902.
14. Gavin LE, Black MM, Minor S, Abel Y, Papas MA, Bentley ME. Young, disadvantaged fathers' involvement with their infants: an ecological perspective. J Adolesc Health. 2002;31(3):266–76.
15. Greenacre P. Problems of overidealization of the analyst and of analysis: their manifestations in the transference and countertransference relationships. Psychoanalytic Study Child. 1966;21:193–212. New York: International Universities Press.
16. Hawkins AJ & Dollahite DC. (Eds.). (1997). Generative fathering: beyond deficit perspectives. Sage Publications, Inc.

17. Howard K, Lefever J, Borkowski J, Whitman T, Kazak AE. Fathers' Influence in the lives of children with adolescent mothers. J Fam Psychol. 2006;20(3):468–76.
18. Kiselica S. When boys become parents: adolescent fatherhood in America. New Brunswick: Rutgers University Press; 2008.
19. Landry D, Forrest J. How old are US fathers? Fam Plan Perspect. 1995;27:159–61.
20. Lewin BD. Dream psychology and the analytic situation. Psychoanal Quart. 1955;24:169–99.
21. Livingston G. Fewer than half of U.S. kids today live in a 'traditional' family. Pew Research Center; 2014. https://www.pewresearch.org/fact-tank/2014/12/22/less-than-half-of-u-s-kids-today-live-in-a-traditional-family/
22. Mahler MS, Gosliner BJ. On symbiotic child psychosis: genetic, dynamic and restitutive aspects. Psychoanalytic Study Child. 1955;10:195–212. Reprinted in *The Selected Papers of Margaret S. Mahler*, vol. 1, eh. 6. New York: Jason Aronson, 1979.
23. Mahler MS. Discussion of Dr. Greenacre's: problems of overidealization of the analyst and of analysis. Unpublished manuscript; 1966 (Abstracted in: *Psychoanalytic Quarterly* 36:637, 1967.)
24. Males M, Chew K. The ages of fathers in California adolescent births, 1993. Am J Public Health. 1996;86(4):565–8.
25. Maravilla B, Cruz CE, Alati. Factors influencing repeated teenage pregnancy: a review and meta-analysis. Am J Obstet Gynecol. 2017;217(5):527–45.e31.
26. Martin JA, Hamilton BE, Osterman MJK, et al. Births: final data for 2015, National vital statistics report; vol 66, no 1. Hyattsville: National Center for Health Statistics; 2017.
27. Maxwell N, Scourfield J, Featherstone B, Holland S, Tolman R. Engaging fathers in child welfare services: a narrative review of recent research evidence. Child Fam Soc Work. 2012;17:160–9. https://doi.org/10.1111/j.1365-2206.2012.00827.x.
28. Mazza C. Young dads: the effects of a parenting program on urban African-American adolescent fathers. Adolescence. 2002;37(148):681–93.
29. MSN.com. 19 Famous young fathers. July 15, 2015. From https://www.msn.com/en-us/lifestyle/family/19-famous-young-fathers/ss-AAd3YgD. Accessed 12 Dec 2018.
30. Panter-Brick C, Burgess A, Eggerman M, McAllister F, Pruett K, & Leckman JF. (2014). Practitioner review: Engaging fathers--recommendations for a game change in parenting interventions based on a systematic review of the global evidence. J Child Psychol Psychiatry, 55(11), 1187–1212. https://doi.org/10.1111/jcpp.12280.
31. Salihu, et al. Assessing the economic impact of paternal involvement: a comparison of the generalized linear model versus decision analysis trees. Matern Child Health J. 2014;18:1380–90.
32. Sarkadi A, Kristiansson R, Oberklaid F, Bremberg S. Fathers' involvement and children's developmental outcomes: a systematic review of longitudinal studies. Acta paediatrica (Oslo, Norway: 1992). 2008;97(2):153–8. https://doi.org/10.1111/j.1651-2227.2007.00572.x.
33. Shrier I, Platt RW. Reducing bias through directed acyclic graphs. BMC Med Res Methodol. 2008;8:70. https://doi.org/10.1186/1471-2288-8-70.
34. Sipsma H, Biello KB, Cole-Lewis H, Kershaw T. Like father, like son: the intergenerational cycle of adolescent fatherhood. Am J Public Health. 2010;100(3):517–24. https://doi.org/10.2105/AJPH.2009.177600.
35. TT Mums. 15 male celebs you had no idea were young dads. October 30, 2017. From https://www.babygaga.com/15-male-celebs-you-had-no-idea-were-young-dads/. Accessed 12 Dec 2018.
36. Winnicott DW. The Child, the Family and the Outside World. Penguin Books, 1964 - Child development - 238 pages.
37. Xie, et al. Predicting teen motherhood and teen fatherhood: individual characteristics and peer affiliations. Soc Dev. 2001;10(4):488–511.

Infant Development and Stigma

6

Jean-Victor P. Wittenberg

Introduction

Outcomes for the group of children of adolescent mothers have been shown to be inferior to outcomes for children of older mothers. There are many explanations for this disparity. It is likely that many different factors act in concert, aggravating or adding to each other and making it difficult to create specific and focused interventions to improve outcomes. It is important to keep in mind that there are teen mothers who do very well in their lives and for whom pregnancy and motherhood distinguish them from their peers. It is clearly the case that some children of teen mothers also do well, but as a group they are at risk.

This chapter continues to expand on the theme that stigma, which often targets teen mothers and babies, causes stress to the mothers and thus indirectly to the babies; it also causes stress directly to the babies in some circumstances. Stigma, acting in multiple ways (see Chap. 3), has been shown to be a stressful experience. These stresses are likely to contribute to the inferior outcomes for the babies, as well as for their adolescent mothers. Considering stress as a pathway to disability can guide designs for prevention and for interventions.

Misinformation and misattributions about teen mothers are the basis of stigma. It is clear that as a group, children of adolescent mothers have higher rates of developmental delays, behavior problems, health problems, mental health problems and substance abuse, higher rates of child protection involvement, early mortality, educational and vocational underachievement, reliance on social support in adulthood, juvenile delinquency and criminality, less life satisfaction and less income than children born to older mothers (e.g., [1, 17, 30, 34, 48]). It is important however, to understand that factors that pre-exist pregnancy and motherhood, such as social

J.-V. P. Wittenberg (✉)
University of Toronto, Toronto, ON, Canada

Hospital for Sick Children, Toronto, ON, Canada
e-mail: jean.wittenberg@sickkids.ca

J.-V. P. Wittenberg et al. (eds.), *Adolescent Pregnancy and Parenting*,
https://doi.org/10.1007/978-3-031-42502-8_6

disadvantage, are more likely to predict these undesirable outcomes than is young maternal age.

One questionable narrative is that young mothers are bad mothers. Some studies have found that teen mothers, as a group, are less responsive, insensitive, more detached, and more likely to be inappropriately intrusive with their babies [20]. Some have described them as more likely to be abusive; at higher risk for psychological and physical aggression; more likely to spank their children; and more likely to be restrictive [33]. These findings are cause for concern but it is also clear that teen mothers are more stressed by their circumstances and by stigma, which are more likely to predict these findings. Alongside multiple reports of increased rates of child maltreatment by teen mothers, however, at least one study found that when other social risk factors were controlled for, there was no evidence for higher rates of maltreatment [10]. Reviews of studies have found that the evidence for an association between young maternal age and child maltreatment is questionable [55] although some studies continue to find a significant association [44]. Studies of adolescent mothering do find a significant association between maltreatment of their children and a history of maltreatment in their own childhoods [54] but the same is true for mothers of all ages [39]. The undesirable outcomes have been shown to be more strongly related to pre-existing factors such as social disadvantage, child maltreatment, developmental trauma, toxic stress, and high levels of adverse childhood experiences (ACEs), in the lives of the teen mothers. Outcomes for children of adolescent mothers are all too often seen as due to maternal age and to very negative attributions about them; there are widely held beliefs that teen mothers are delinquent, promiscuous, impulsive, unintelligent, that they are bad mothers, etc. The finding that the undesirable outcomes relate more strongly to disadvantage and stress than to the age of the mothers, is often overlooked or disregarded [1]. Ignoring what research has shown to be the root causes of the unfavorable outcomes, these false beliefs further stigmatize young mothers, worsening the outcomes for the mother and child.

Stigma clearly stresses these mothers and babies in many ways and at many times in their lives. There are higher rates of teen pregnancies in minority groups that are stigmatized, thus disadvantage predicts teen pregnancy. Weiman et al. [72] found that teen mothers are aware of stigma in pregnancy. Zeiders et al. [74] found that cumulative stresses of discrimination and acculturalization measured from pregnancy to 2 years after delivery, affected not only the mothers but also the grandmothers in a Mexican American population. This finding may be of relevance as grandmothers are often primary caregivers to children of single mothers. Their relationships with their daughters (i.e., the teen mothers) may become stressed because of the stigma and we know that when the grandmother-mother relationship is stressed and conflictual, the outcomes for mothers and children is significantly compromised. These conflictual relationships interfere with the capacity of teen mothers to develop a sense of competence as mothers – a sense of competence that protects the health and development of their children [60]. These cumulative stresses are associated with adverse developmental, behavioral, and educational outcomes in the children at age 5 years [74].

The population of teen mothers is a vulnerable population, composed of many individuals whose lives have been disadvantaged and stressed, whose ability to regulate their emotions and behavior, to use executive function and to make adaptive decisions has been compromised by those stresses and adverse childhood experiences. Steele et al. [67] found that there was a clear association between women's exposure to adverse childhood experiences (ACEs) and their parental distress as mothers. Nonetheless many teen mothers, even many who have endured disadvantage, are capable individuals who have been shown to become able to make significant progress in their lives subsequent to the birth of their babies [46, 62]. Stigma adds to their burden of stress whether they are more or less capable, and thus is likely to adversely impact outcomes for themselves, their babies and children.

Healthy Development in Infancy and Early Childhood

Freud defined mental health for adults as the capacity to love and work ([23] -https://www.thecanadianencyclopedia.ca/en/article/mental-health). Others including Winnicott [73] added the capacity to play or to be creative. In the present day, having the advantage of a huge knowledge base addressing infant development, we would include the following as components of mental health in infancy and childhood:

- being able to engage positively with caregivers and others, both children and adults;
- being able to regulate feelings and behavior;
- being able to adapt to changes and to different situations;
- being able to explore the world;
- being able to learn, develop and grow;
- being able to play and use creativity.

The absence of any of these capacities marks a significant deficit in mental health and development. Within each capacity, there are many variations which can be healthy and others that limit capacity. There is a wide consensus that healthy development and even survival, depend on environmental supports beginning with the immediate family and extending out to the community, even to global issues such as pollution, international conflict, poverty, etc. [61]. We depend on relationships with each other for biological needs (shelter, food, procreation, etc.), emotional needs (emotion regulation, intimacy, etc.), social needs (learning how to exist in the social groups within which humans live), and cognitive needs (stimulation, education, etc.) [28]

Earlier theories suggested divisions between physical and mental, nature and nurture, biological and experiential but our knowledge base now clearly shows that they are interdependent; development of biological systems influences our psychology and our experiences shape our biological systems. Each acts on the other in an interdependent line of development.

We have also learned about the significance of development beginning in our earliest years. Shonkoff et al. [61] drew connections between health and its dependency on biology, the physical and social environments.

> Beginning prenatally, continuing through infancy, and extending into childhood and beyond, development is driven by an ongoing, inextricable interaction between biology (as defined by genetic predispositions) and ecology (as defined by the social and physical environment).

Those interactions between the fetus, baby, young child, and the environment can be differentiated as supportive or stressful. Not all stress is damaging. It can spur development in adaptive ways if it can be mastered, when it does not tax the stress management systems excessively. If a child is well prepared and well supported, stress can have some impact, but recovery and even growth are possible. When it overwhelms the child's capacity to regulate herself, stress is traumatizing and can lead to PTSD in infants and young children as much as in older children, youth and adults. In fact, PTSD often is underdiagnosed and overlooked or dismissed at younger ages [57].

Stress is also damaging if it is excessively challenging and occurs for prolonged periods or repeatedly. Shonkoff and his colleagues [61] defined toxic stress as that which challenges the stress response system excessively; it leads to serious adverse consequences. Felitti et al. [18] found that ACEs were associated with problems of health and development across the lifespan. ACEs are stress-inducing experiences. Disorders associated with high exposure to ACEs include psychiatric disorders, cognitive disorders, relational difficulties, addictive problems, a very wide range of physical disorders, etc. One very relevant finding in these studies has been that higher levels of ACEs are found in both the mothers' lives and in their babies' lives from early infancy [43]. The consequences of the teenage mother's early childhood stresses explain the relatively poor functioning of their children. They remain vulnerable to stress in childhood, adolescence, and adulthood. Stigmatizing social attitudes add to their stress burden and compromise their functioning.

Attachment Theory Attachment theory, perhaps the most influential theory underpinning our understanding of infancy, is a theory of relationships and of stress regulation. Attachment classifications reflect an internalized strategy for dealing with and regulating stress, learned through relationships in the first 12–18 months of life. Specifically, attachment is conceptualized as a system for regulating the stress associated with feelings of insecurity in infants. Secure attachment is associated with better social functioning, better learning, better physical and mental health and less psychopathology in children, teens, and adults [65, 68, 69]. Attachment classifications have been directly connected to physiological reactions to stress [24]. Insecure attachment (avoidant, resistant or disorganized classifications) is associated with less effective strategies for dealing with stress and less socially supportive relationships with caregivers. Caregivers of infants with avoidant or resistant attachment classifications are described as dismissive of expressions of negative affect or inconsistently responsive to negative affect in their infants. Disorganized attachment is associated with disruptive and/or frightening caregiver responses to infants. Maternal experiences and expressions of stress tend to be transmitted to the baby. The FR behaviors described by Main and Hesse [40] and the disruptive behaviors described by Lyons-Ruth et al. [38] are associated with disorganized attachment and can be seen as behaviors that increase when caregivers are stressed.

Some studies find higher levels of insecurity in infants of teen mothers (e.g., [36]) whereas other studies report no elevation of rates of insecurity [2, 16]. When a teen mother reported low stress and satisfaction with social support at 10 months, her baby was more likely to show secure attachment. Teen mothers of insecure babies report higher levels of stress and lower levels of social support compared to peers. This may speak to the needs that adolescents have for social supports to help them regulate their own levels of stress.

Overall, we see that mothers who are more highly stressed tend to transmit suboptimal stress management systems to their babies. Unfortunately, these are the babies who need highly functioning stress management capacity as they are more likely to encounter stress on a day-to-day basis. We postulate that this is an inflection point in the development of infants and children of teen mothers: (1) many teen mothers come from a disadvantaged and stressed population; (2) their experiences of stress leave them vulnerable to dysfunction in the face of stress in the future; (3) they are highly likely to be targets of stigma; (4) stigma increases their stress levels; (5) their babies and children experience those higher levels of stress; (6) these children are predisposed to adverse outcomes as described in the ACE and attachment literatures.

Stress Before and During Pregnancy

Preconception Stress Much has been found about stress in pregnancy; we are now learning that stress affects parents and their future offspring even before conception. Lane et al. [32] refer to stress affecting germ cells then leaving a mark on the yet to be conceived zygote. Fluid in mother's ovaries and fallopian tubes are affected by maternal nutritional, metabolic, and inflammatory factors. Stress is repeatedly associated with inflammatory changes [35]. The embryo is exquisitely sensitive to these influences and adapts, as it were, to mother's external environment. These adaptations may be helpful to the infant when she is born, or they may be limiting and maladaptive.

In fathers, obesity, history of smoking and exposure to occupational chemicals are associated with changes in their children. These findings are particularly relevant to babies of teen parents as these parents are often highly stressed, have higher rates of unhealthy living habits including smoking and are more likely to be exposed to environmental toxins (Shonkoff et al. 2021). Teen fathers, like teen mothers, are more likely to come from disadvantaged backgrounds and thus to be more stressed.

Prenatal stressfulness in fathers is independently associated with possible problems in regulatory functioning in their babies [22].

Mothers who are likely to have developed compromised stress management responses are more likely to pass that on to their babies. Their babies show signs of stress difficulties very early in their lives. There is significant evidence that early traumatic experiences in mothers predict stressed responsiveness in their young babies. Women who were witnesses to interpersonal violence in their own childhoods have babies who show evidence of altered stress responses in the first days and months of life [39, 51].

Stress in Pregnancy The impact of stress in pregnancy is lasting and has been shown to be associated with changes into adolescence. Offspring whose mothers reported anxiety or depression in pregnancy showed blunted cortisol responses as adolescents. Hamada and Matthews [26] suggested that these outcomes were mediated by changes in epigenetic modifications. This is particularly relevant to the population of adolescent mothers who are often children of stressed adolescent mothers themselves. The stresses of one generation are communicated to and visited on subsequent generations.

Pregnant and mothering adolescents clearly experience stigma [72] and as a result have elevated levels of stress. Many, but not all, teen pregnancies are unintended or unwanted. Unintended and unwanted pregnancies are associated with stress that can be transmitted to babies, sometimes before birth, in several ways. Unintended pregnancy is associated with depression in pregnancy and in the postpartum period. Shaming, stigmatizing responses from others when a young woman is pregnant are highly stress inducing. This kind of stigma is associated with social isolation and deprivation, both of which are likely to incur further deleterious outcomes to the young mother and her child.

Osok et al. [50] described a number of mechanisms by which stigma increases the stressful experiences of teen mothers in Kenya. They wrote that pregnant adolescents face four major areas of challenges related to social and cultural values:

- *Depression, anxiety, and stress around the pregnancy* – All three experiences lead to elevated levels of stress hormones and transmission of stress to the unborn baby. There is clear evidence of associated physiological and epigenetic changes. Social and cultural norms around the world reduce the status of adolescent girls who are pregnant. This stigma undoubtedly invokes stress for the pregnant teens and makes it more likely that they will experience depression and anxiety.
- *Denial of the pregnancy* – Denial of pregnancy can occur as a result of several factors. These may include a lack of self-awareness, perhaps not surprising in disadvantaged adolescent girls. It may be influenced by developmental and psychological struggles, again not surprising in this disadvantaged population. Finally, it may be strongly influenced by the adolescent's wish not to be pregnant and fear of disapproval from those around her including her parents; i.e., stigma. (Of course, like the other factors mentioned here, this will not be the case for all

teens who become pregnant; some choose to be pregnant and welcome the baby as do their parents or other supports. They are likely to feel less stressed.)

- *Lack of basic needs provisions and care* – Pregnant teens and teens who have babies, especially those who do not receive support from their families, are likely to be poor. They may have food and housing insecurity. They may have to accept arrangements that are suboptimal; some living arrangements may expose them to maltreatment. They may struggle to get social supports. In the process of arranging to get social supports, be it from family or from social agencies, they are likely to be exposed to critical and demeaning attitudes, i.e., stigma. Poverty and lack of healthy nutrition, before pregnancy, during pregnancy and afterwards are associated with health problems, developmental problems difficulties with executive function, learning problems and relationship problems for the babies as they grow. These will continue to impose stress throughout the lives of these children.
- *Restricted educational or livelihood opportunities for personal development post-pregnancy* – Loss of opportunities for improvement and loss of hope for improvement in life leads to fewer resources, fewer chances to learn how to address challenges and a greater sense of despair.

Exposure to maternal stress during pregnancy has been shown to be associated with negative effects in babies [3, 6, 11, 37, 53]. At birth babies have lower birthweight, lower APGAR scores and are more likely to need resuscitation at birth. Excessive stress in pregnant women leads to epigenetic changes in the placenta, in the brain and in peripheral tissues [41]. All are associated with adverse effects on both physical and mental health for the baby. In infancy and childhood, they have problems with stress management, higher rates of psychopathology, and difficulties with executive function. Monk et al. [47] found an epigenetic effect on the placenta that affects placental metabolism of cortisol, which in turn is associated with subsequent psychopathology in children.

Chan et al. [8] reviewed the impact and mechanisms of stress in pregnancy on neurodevelopment. Stressful challenges can include starvation, immune challenges, and social or psychological stressors. They describe how stresses for the mother lead to changes in epigenetic programming of the fetus. The effect is to transmit stress as experienced by the mother to the fetus. Key developmental signals are altered throughout the pregnancy. The HPA axis of the developing fetus is programmed to expect and respond to heightened levels of stress. This dysregulation is associated with multiple disorders that appear subsequently including autism, schizophrenia, affective disorders, and ADHD.

The population of pregnant teens and teen mothers is at high risk for stress-related disorders. Maternal depressed mood in pregnancy is more common in adolescents and is associated with epigenetic changes altering infant HPA stress reactivity [49]. Rates of mental health disorders, addiction, and substance abuse are higher in individuals ages 15–24 years [52] and are associated with higher rates of unintended pregnancies [9]. There is evidence that the use of substances in pregnancy is associated with an epigenetically mediated higher rate of addiction in their offspring [70].

Sex of the fetus and timing of stresses in pregnancy have influences such that males are reported to be put more at risk for schizophrenia and ASD especially if stress is in the first and second trimesters. Females are reported to be at higher risk for affective disorders when their mothers are exposed to stress in early pregnancy. Late pregnancy stress is associated with cognitive difficulties and ADHD [8].

There is very good evidence that to avoid inflicting damage on unborn babies and children preventive health initiatives that support their parents are necessary.

Stress in Infancy Stress need not be an undesirable or adverse experience. It can provide opportunities to develop skills and capacities in many realms including self-regulation, interpersonal relationships, and even immunological responses (e.g., [42]). Healthy degrees of stress can enhance immunoprotective functions whereas chronic stress (toxic stress) tends to suppress immune responses or exacerbate pathological immune responses [13]. The human infant has few ways of dealing with stress and depends on her/his caregivers to modulate stress and its impact. Just as with immune function, excessive stress or stress that is not socially regulated (i.e., buffered) can have very deleterious effects on infants' development and mental health [61].

Having adult caregivers who help infants modulate their responses to stress predicts positive vs. negative impacts (e.g., [21, 61]). Infants show significantly higher physiological responses to stress in the absence of an attachment figure [25]. When infants were stressed, their ability to learn and function optimally was compromised; they lost cognitive flexibility and performed in rigid manners [59].

There are a range of factors that can cause stress for infants, and infants who come from disadvantaged backgrounds are more likely to be stressed. The ACE studies and studies of toxic stress clearly link stressful experiences in early childhood with serious physical and mental health problems at all ages and with shortened lifespan [19]. Parents who have difficulty managing stress are more likely to transmit stress to their babies.

Bidirectional Influences When babies are born with higher demands for care, parents are more likely to feel increased stress. Babies of teen mothers are more likely to be born with conditions such as prematurity or low birth weight [11], that make them more challenging to parent. Behavior problems in children and parental stress have been noted to exacerbate each other. Hastings et al. [27] provided evidence of a bidirectional relationship whereby increased maternal stress leads to increased child behavior problems and child behavior problems lead to increased maternal stress over time, independent of maternal mental health.

As described in the chapter on adolescent development, teen mothers are particularly vulnerable to stress. Babies clearly need support and protection from undue stress. Thus, they form a dyad likely to have serious difficulty managing stress and are likely to each challenge the other's adaptation.

Thirteen- to eighteen-year-old females are at highest risk among adolescents for PTSD [45]. Infants and young children can also be traumatized and often that diagnosis has been overlooked for the young age group [57]. It seems likely that when an adolescent mother is traumatized the risk of PTSD is also higher in their infants and toddlers. Unfortunately, they can become triggers for each other; distress in one triggers a pathological stress response in the other. This interactional vulnerability can prolong or even defeat recovery [56, 58].

Social Supports There is evidence that many of the problems seen in the children of teen mothers can be mitigated by post-natal experiences. The same is true of many other populations such as infants who spend time in the NICU at birth [5]. The quality of the babies' experiences in the post-natal period is determined by many factors including their mothers' degree of comfort and confidence in caring for the baby. Mother's comfort is determined by her sense of social support. Teens are particularly susceptible to the stress-inducing effects of social interactions (e.g., [15]). Thus, providing these young families a sense of support becomes particularly salient when designing appropriate post-natal interventions.

Many infants of teen mothers function within normal ranges on developmental assessments and social-emotional measures in the first year; however, social-emotional difficulties become apparent by the end of the first year and delays in intellectual functioning thereafter [74]. Infants who show delays are more likely to come from homes where there are more stresses: poverty, fewer learning materials, maternal depression, and conflict [29]. Even when there are early stresses, supportive family environments predict better emotional and cognitive development.

Aizer et al. [1] found teen mothers' choice of fathers had a significant impact; fathers' low education levels and low cognitive scores were associated with more adverse outcomes for children. These fathers have less to invest, in terms of human capital as well as financial support, in their offspring and that is likely to affect child outcomes.

Poverty Adolescent parents tend to be poor. They have fewer toys and access to fewer programs for infant and child stimulation. The absence of toys and programs reduces the number and duration of parent–child interactions. Teen parents are seen as having less patience or motivation to engage their babies; the absence of toys may even further reduce their interactions. Babies who are deprived of supportive, interactive and regulating interactions are slower developmentally; they are less likely to be school-ready. They are more likely to be seen by teachers as less capable and less intelligent. [29].

Interventions

Evaluations have found that some interventions are helpful, but much remains to be done to ascertain what works and what does not [31]. Careful evaluations will depend on appropriate comparisons and controls. In the past, research was strongly influenced by stigmatizing attitudes. Teen mothers were compared to teens who had not experienced the same disadvantages. Researchers concluded that the teens were doing badly when in some cases they did better than appropriately selected controls [46, 62]. Studies emphasize the need to base both preventive and therapeutic interventions on knowledge of context and etiology, biological, psychological, and developmental implications, as well as on clinically significant changes. Thus reports to date require careful evaluation of bias before applying their findings to interventions.

Social disadvantage is the most influential predictor of teen pregnancy and of undesirable outcomes for both adolescent mothers and their babies. Social supports and psychotherapeutic interventions can lead to better outcomes but cannot compensate for social determinants of health that have left marks on the mothers (and fathers) and on the babies from their early years. Stigma is a significant contributor to social disadvantage. Social disadvantage directly affects both mothers and babies, and the effect of disadvantage is multiplied when the impact on mothers is transmitted to the babies. Improvement depends on changes in policies at many levels, in practices in many domains including the offices of healthcare professionals and in social attitudes. It has been shown that we can change social attitudes. For example, smoking tobacco has been reduced by public campaign (e.g., [14]) as has use of seat belts in motor vehicles [71]. The Black Lives Matter campaign has reduced police killings [7].

Nonetheless reviews have found that there can be significant changes albeit with small effect size, because of interventions that target repeat pregnancy, health in pregnancy and low birthweight of newborns, maternal education, and employment [64]. There is no doubt that sex education and access to contraception are the most effective interventions to reduce teen pregnancy [66].

Specialized programs adapted to the needs of teen mothers and their babies tend to have multiple components (e.g., case management, healthcare services for mothers and babies, parent counseling and support, education, etc.). They have shown associations with improvement in rates of child abuse, well-baby visits and rates of immunization, as well as identification and referrals for concerns about developmental delays [12, 44]. There have been findings that programs adapted for teen mothers are associated with improvement in substance abuse and improvement in symptoms of depression. There is some evidence that these maternal improvements were associated with fewer externalizing and internalizing symptoms in their children [63]. A program adapted specifically to the culture of native American teen mothers found positive benefits in children's externalizing, internalizing, and dysregulation symptoms [4].

The effectiveness of parenting interventions is less clear. A review of meta-analyses of intervention studies [64] found no evidence that interventions improved appropriate developmental expectations of children, empathic awareness, the undesirableness of corporal punishment, and parent–child role reversal in teen mothers. There was some evidence to support improvements in parent–child teaching interaction and in measures of parent child relationship. This is a very important finding needing much more research and is considered further in the chapter on interventions.

Conclusions

When it is overwhelming or when it is chronic and taxes the stress management systems of the individual, stress can have damaging effects. Stigma exerts stress in many ways. Optimal health, educational and social benefits will accrue when we provide support rather than stress for children and families. This is true for all mothers and babies but perhaps especially for adolescent mothers and their babies. Providing support will require changes in policy at many levels, changes in social and professional attitudes in many social domains and perhaps most salient, recognition of the damage we create when we hold stigmatizing attitudes. Prevention is clearly preferable to repair. Interventions to help disadvantaged populations cannot entirely compensate for damage that has been inflicted earlier. Supporting mothers and babies helps us all.

References

1. Aizer A, Devereaux P, Salvanes K. Grandparents, Moms, or Dads? Why children of teen mothers do worse in life. J Hum Resour. 2020; 1019-10524R2.
2. Andreozzi L, Flanagan P, Seifer R, Brunner S, Lester B. Attachment classifications among 18-month-old children of adolescent mothers. Arch Pediatr Adolesc Med. 2002;156(1):20–6.
3. Azar R, Paquette D, Zoccolillo M, Baltzer F, Tremblay RE. The association of major depression, conduct disorder, and maternal overcontrol with a failure to show a cortisol buffered response in 4-month-old infants of teenage mothers. Biol Psychiatry. 2007;62(6):573–9.
4. Barlow A, Mullany B, Neault N, Goklish N, Billy T, Hastings R, et al. Paraprofessional-delivered home-visiting intervention for American Indian teen mothers and children: 3-year outcomes from a randomized controlled trial. Am J Psychiatr. 2015;172(2):154–62.
5. Benzies KM, Magill-Evans JE, Hayden KA, Ballantyne M. Key components of early intervention programs for preterm infants and their parents: a systematic review and meta-analysis. BMC Pregnancy Childbirth. 2013;13(1):1–15.
6. Blair C, Granger DA, Willoughby M, Mills-Koonce R, Cox M, Greenberg MT, et al. Salivary cortisol mediates effects of poverty and parenting on executive functions in early childhood. Child Dev. 2011;82(6):1970–84.
7. Campbell T. Black Lives Matter's effect on police lethal use-of-force. 2021; Available at SSRN.
8. Chan JC, Nugent BM, Bale TL. Parental advisory: maternal and paternal stress can impact offspring neurodevelopment. Biol Psychiatry. 2018;83(10):886–94.
9. Connery HS, Albright BB, Rodolico JM. Adolescent substance use and unplanned pregnancy: strategies for risk reduction. Obstet Gynecol Clin. 2014;41(2):191–203.
10. Coren E, Barlow J. Individual and group-based parenting programmes for improving psychosocial outcomes for teenage parents and their children. Cochrane Database Syst Rev. 2001

11. Coussons-Read ME. Effects of prenatal stress on pregnancy and human development: mechanisms and pathways. Obstet Med. 2013;6(2):52–7.
12. Cox JE, Harris SK, Conroy K, Engelhart T, Vyavaharkar A, Federico A, Woods ER. A parenting and life skills intervention for teen mothers: a randomized controlled trial. Pediatrics. 2019;143(3):e20182303.
13. Dhabhar FS. Effects of stress on immune function: the good, the bad, and the beautiful. Immunol Res. 2014;58(2):193–210.
14. Durkin SJ, Biener L, Wakefield MA. Effects of different types of antismoking ads on reducing disparities in smoking cessation among socioeconomic subgroups. Am J Public Health. 2009;99(12):2217–23.
15. Eiland L, Romeo RD. Stress and the developing adolescent brain. Neuroscience. 2013;249:162–71.
16. Emery J, Paquette D, Bigras M. Factors predicting attachment patterns in infants of adolescent mothers. J Fam Stud. 2008;14(1):65–90.
17. Fagan J, Lee Y. Explaining the association between adolescent parenting and preschoolers' school readiness: a risk perspective. J Community Psychol. 2013;41(6):692–708.
18. Felitti VJ, Anda RF, Nordenberg D, Williamson DF, Spitz AM, Edwards V, Marks JS. Relationship of childhood abuse and household dysfunction to many of the leading causes of death in adults: the adverse childhood experiences (ACE) study. Am J Prev Med. 1998b;14(4):245–58.
19. Felitti VJ, Anda RF, Nordenberg D, Williamson DF. Adverse childhood experiences and health outcomes in adults: the Ace study. J Fam Consum Sci. 1998a;90(3):31.
20. Flaherty SC, Sadler LS. A review of attachment theory in the context of adolescent parenting. J Pediatr Health Care. 2011;25(2):114–21.
21. Franke HA. Toxic stress: effects, prevention and treatment. Children. 2014;1(3):390–402.
22. Gao M, Brown MA, Neff D, Crowell SE, Conradt E. Prenatal paternal stress predicts infant parasympathetic functioning above and beyond maternal prenatal stress. J Reprod Infant Psychol. 2021;40:1–14.
23. Goodman JT. 2016. https://www.thecanadianencyclopedia.ca/en/article/mental-health
24. Gunnar MR, Brodersen L, Nachmias M, Buss K, Rigatuso J. Stress reactivity and attachment security. Dev Psychobiol. 1996;29(3):191–204.
25. Gunnar MR, Hostinar CE. The social buffering of the hypothalamic–pituitary–adrenocortical axis in humans: Developmental and experiential determinants. Soc Neurosci. 2015;10(5):479–88.
26. Hamada H, Matthews SG. Prenatal programming of stress responsiveness and behaviours: progress and perspectives. J Neuroendocrinol. 2019;31(3):e12674.
27. Hastings RP, Daley D, Burns C, Beck A. Maternal distress and expressed emotion: cross-sectional and longitudinal relationships with behavior problems of children with intellectual disabilities. Am J Ment Retard. 2006;111(1):48–61.
28. Hertzman C, Boyce T. How experience gets under the skin to create gradients in developmental health. Annu Rev Public Health. 2010;31:329–47.
29. Jahromi LB, Umana-Taylor AJ, Updegraff KA, Zeiders KH. Trajectories of developmental functioning among children of adolescent mothers; factors associated with risk of delay. Amer J Intellect Dev Disabil. 2016 July;121(4):346–63.
30. Jutte DP, Roos NP, Brownell MD, Briggs G, MacWilliam L, Roos LL. The ripples of adolescent motherhood: social, educational, and medical outcomes for children of teen and prior teen mothers. Acad Pediatr. 2010;10(5):293–301.
31. Lachance CR, Burrus BB, Scott AR. Building an evidence base to inform interventions for pregnant and parenting adolescents: a call for rigorous evaluation. Am J Public Health. 2012;102(10):1826–32.
32. Lane M, Robker RL, Robertson SA. Parenting from before conception. Science. 2014;345(6198):756–60.
33. Lee Y, Guterman NB. Young mother–father dyads and maternal harsh parenting behavior. Child Abuse Negl. 2010;34(11):874–85.

34. Lipman EL, Georgiades K, Boyle MH. Young adult outcomes of children born to teen mothers: effects of being born during their teen or later years. J Am Acad Child Adolesc Psychiatry. 2011;50(3):232–41.
35. Liu YZ, Wang YX, Jiang CL. Inflammation: the common pathway of stress-related diseases. Front Hum Neurosci. 2017;11:316.
36. Lounds JJ, Borkowski JG, Whitman TL, Maxwell SE, Weed K. Adolescent parenting and attachment during infancy and early childhood. Parent Sci Pract. 2005;5(1):91–118.
37. Lupien SJ, McEwen BS, Gunnar MR, Heim C. Effects of stress throughout the lifespan on the brain, behaviour and cognition. Nat Rev Neurosci. 2009;10(6):434–45.
38. Lyons-Ruth K, Bronfman E, Parsons E. Chapter IV. Maternal frightened, frightening, or atypical behavior and disorganized infant attachment patterns. Monogr Soc Res Child Dev. 1999;64(3):67–96.
39. Madigan S, Cyr C, Eirich R, Fearon RP, Ly A, Rash C, et al. Testing the cycle of maltreatment hypothesis: Meta-analytic evidence of the intergenerational transmission of child maltreatment. Dev Psychopathol. 2019;31(1):23–51.
40. Main M, Hesse E. Parents' unresolved traumatic experiences are related to infant disorganized attachment status: Is frightened and/or frightening parental behavior the linking mechanism? The University of Chicago Press; 1990.
41. Maniam J, Antoniadis C, Morris MJ. Early-life stress, HPA axis adaptation, and mechanisms contributing to later health outcomes. Front Endocrinol. 2014;5:73.
42. Masten AS. Resilience theory and research on children and families: past, present, and promise. J Fam Theory Rev. 2018;10(1):12–31.
43. McDonnell CG, Valentino K. Intergenerational effects of childhood trauma: evaluating pathways among maternal ACEs, perinatal depressive symptoms, and infant outcomes. Child Maltreatment. 2016;21(4):317–26.
44. McHugh MT, Kvernland A, Palusci VJ. An adolescent parents' programme to reduce child abuse. Child Abuse Rev. 2017;26(3):184–95.
45. Merikangas, K. R., He, J. P., Burstein, M., Swanson, S. A., Avenevoli, S., Cui, L., … & Swendsen, J. (2010). Lifetime prevalence of mental disorders in US adolescents: results from the National Comorbidity Survey Replication–Adolescent Supplement (NCS-A). J Am Acad Child Adolesc Psychiatry, 49(10), 980-989.
46. Mollborn S. Teenage Mothers Today: What We Know and How It Matters. Child Dev Perspect. 2017;11(1):63–9. https://doi.org/10.1111/cdep.12205. Epub 2016 Nov 7. PMID: 28533814; PMCID: PMC5438165.
47. Monk C, Feng T, Lee S, Krupska I, Champagne FA, Tycko B. Distress during pregnancy: epigenetic regulation of placenta glucocorticoid-related genes and fetal neurobehavior. Am J Psychiatr. 2016;173(7):705–13.
48. Oberlander SE, Black MM. African American adolescent mothers' early caregiving involvement and children's behavior and academic performance at age 7. J Clin Child Adolesc Psychol. 2011;40(5):756–64.
49. Oberlander TF, Weinberg J, Papsdorf M, Grunau R, Misri S, Devlin AM. Prenatal exposure to maternal depression, neonatal methylation of human glucocorticoid receptor gene (NR3C1) and infant cortisol stress responses. Epigenetics. 2008;3(2):97–106.
50. Osok J, Kigamwa P, Huang KY, Grote N, Kumar M. Adversities and mental health needs of pregnant adolescents in Kenya: identifying interpersonal, practical, and cultural barriers to care. BMC Womens Health. 2018;18(1):1–18.
51. Parade SH, Newland RP, Bublitz MH, Stroud LR. Maternal witness to intimate partner violence during childhood and prenatal family functioning alter newborn cortisol reactivity. Stress. 2019;22(2):190–9.
52. Pearson C, Janz T, Ali J. Mental and substance use disorders in Canada. Statistics Canada; 2013.
53. Ponirakis A, Susman EJ, Stifter CA. Negative emotionality and cortisol during adolescent pregnancy and its effects on infant health and autonomic nervous system reactivity. Dev Psychobiol. 1998;33(2):163–74.

54. Putnam-Hornstein E, Cederbaum JA, King B, Eastman AL, Trickett PK. A population-level and longitudinal study of adolescent mothers and intergenerational maltreatment. Am J Epidemiol. 2015;181(7):496–503.
55. Scannapieco M, Connell-Carrick K. Correlates of child maltreatment among adolescent mothers with young children. J Evid Inform Soc Work. 2016;13(1):59–75.
56. Scheeringa MS. Treating PTSD in preschoolers: a clinical guide. Guilford Publications; 2015.
57. Scheeringa MS, Myers L, Putnam FW, Zeanah CH. Diagnosing PTSD in early childhood: an empirical assessment of four approaches. J Trauma Stress. 2012;25(4):359–67.
58. Scheeringa MS, Myers L, Putnam FW, Zeanah CH. Maternal factors as moderators or mediators of PTSD symptoms in very young children: a two-year prospective study. J Fam Violence. 2015;30(5):633–42.
59. Seehagen S, Schneider S, Rudolph J, Ernst S, Zmyj N. Stress impairs cognitive flexibility in infants. Proc Natl Acad Sci. 2015;112(41):12882–6.
60. Sellers K, Black MM, Boris NW, Oberlander SE, Myers L. Adolescent mothers' relationships with their own mothers: impact on parenting outcomes. J Fam Psychol. 2011;25(1):117.
61. Shonkoff JP, Garner AS, Siegel BS, Dobbins MI, Earls MF, McGuinn L, et al. The lifelong effects of early childhood adversity and toxic stress. Pediatrics. 2012;129(1):e232–46.
62. SmithBattle L. Reframing the risks and losses of teen mothering. MCN Am J Mater Child Nurs. 2009;34(2):122–8.
63. SmithBattle L, Freed P. Teen mothers' mental health. MCN Am J Matern Child Nurs. 2016;41(1):31–6.
64. SmithBattle L, Punsuwun S, Phengnum W. An umbrella review of qualitative research on teen mothering. West J Nurs Res. 2017;43(5):478–88.
65. Sroufe LA. Attachment and development: a prospective, longitudinal study from birth to adulthood. Attach Hum Dev. 2005;7(4):349–67.
66. Stanger-Hall KF, Hall DW. Abstinence-only education and teen pregnancy rates: why we need comprehensive sex education in the US. PLoS One. 2011;6(10):e24658.
67. Steele H, Bate J, Steele M, Dube SR, Danskin K, Knafo H, Nikitiades A, Bonuck K, Meissner P, & Murphy A. Adverse childhood experiences, poverty, and parenting stress. Canadian Journal of Behavioural Science / Revue canadienne des sciences du comportement. 2016;48(1):32–8. https://doi.org/10.1037/cbs0000034.
68. Taubner S, White LO, Zimmermann J, Fonagy P, Nolte T. Attachment-related mentalization moderates the relationship between psychopathic traits and proactive aggression in adolescence. J Abnorm Child Psychol. 2013;41(6):929–38.
69. Thompson R. Early attachment and later development: familiar questions, new answers. In: Handbook of Attachment. New York: Guilford; 2015.
70. Vassoler FM, Sadri-Vakili G. Mechanisms of transgenerational inheritance of addictive-like behaviors. Neuroscience. 2014;264:198–206.
71. Vasudevan V, Nambisan SS, Singh AK, Pearl T. Effectiveness of media and enforcement campaigns in increasing seat belt usage rates in a state with a secondary seat belt law. Traffic Inj Prev. 2009;10(4):330–9. https://doi.org/10.1080/15389580902995190. PMID: 19593709.
72. Wiemann CM, Rickert VI, Berenson AB, Volk RJ. Are pregnant adolescents stigmatized by pregnancy? J Adolesc Health. 2005;36(4):352-e1.
73. Winnicott DW. The family and individual development. London: Routledge; 2012.
74. Zeiders KH, Umaña-Taylor AJ, Jahromi LB, Updegraff KA, White RM. Discrimination and acculturation stress: a longitudinal study of children's well-being from prenatal development to 5 years of age. J Dev Behav Pediatr. 2016;37(7):557–64.

Interventions Supporting and Empowering Pregnant and Parenting Adolescents

7

Liwei L. Hua

Introduction

Although births to adolescent mothers have been declining since peaking in 1991, there were still 171,674 births to adolescents 15–19 years old in 2019 [24]. Repeat pregnancies, defined as those occurring within 24 months of a previous pregnancy, also occur in about 1 in 6 adolescent mothers [25]. Abundant data indicate that pregnant and parenting adolescents are at risk for school dropout; domestic violence; mental health disorders, including depression and suicidal ideation; and living in poverty [14–16, 20, 33]. Their children are at risk of experiencing abuse/neglect, being raised by a single parent or in foster care, lower school achievement, dropping out of high school, and becoming adolescent parents themselves [33]. As we have argued in the preceding chapters, much of this dismal scenario is actually due to psychosocial risk factors that persist prior to, during, and after pregnancy. Appropriately designed supports and services can improve outcomes for teen parents and their children.

Despite bleak outcomes for some adolescents, adolescent pregnancy and parenting can be an empowering and motivating experience, as we saw in the first person accounts in the chapter, *The Voices of Lived Experience*. This is especially true when young people are provided with the necessary supports and resources to encourage self-sufficiency [37]. We know that inherent resilience, parental/school support, and growing up with parents/guardians who stressed the importance of completing school are all factors associated with improved outcomes for both parents and children [4]. Programs that are designed with these factors in mind can support and empower teen parents. These programs can be broadly categorized as (1) school-based services, (2) home visiting programs, (3) community outreach programs, (4) medical home models, and (5) coparenting groups.

L. L. Hua (✉)
South Bend Clinic, South Bend, IN, USA

J.-V. P. Wittenberg et al. (eds.), *Adolescent Pregnancy and Parenting*,
https://doi.org/10.1007/978-3-031-42502-8_7

Prenatal and Postnatal Care

Prenatal and postnatal care for pregnant adolescents and their babies are essential, but adolescents are less likely than older women to receive care in the early stages of pregnancy. Lack of care is associated with the same risk factors that are associated with unplanned pregnancies: substance use, low income, minority status. Lacking knowledge, living in a rural area, not having transportation, having a poor support system, and experiencing stigma can interfere with accessing care [22]. However, pregnancy can serve as the initial opportunity to become engaged in comprehensive healthcare services [20]. It is crucial for providers to recognize that the needs of pregnant adolescents differ from those of older women. Like all patients, teens receiving services need good communication with their health care providers and clear explanations. Pregnant teens also need respectful versus judgmental providers, and they need to be engaged as partners in decision-making. Attitudes of providers are crucial as they can make teens feel demeaned or criticized. When asked about their experiences, adolescents report being questioned about why they were having babies at their age, being interrogated about their partners, and having decisions made about their deliveries or postnatal care without their say [8, 41]. Alternatively, positive experiences with healthcare during pregnancy can not only improve the health of the mother and child, but have an impact on future healthcare seeking behaviors.

Clinical guidelines have been published specifically for adolescent prenatal and postnatal care. They emphasize the importance of routine and repeated screening for conditions that are common in this population, including mood disorders and substance abuse, intimate partner violence, and sexually transmitted diseases [10, 32]. They also recommend supporting the involvement of fathers, and support for breastfeeding and long-acting contraception post-partum. They cite evidence for the superiority of multidisciplinary care. They stress that prenatal care and childbirth education designed for the typical population are unlikely to best serve the pregnant adolescent, and advocate for culturally competent care. Such competence must take into account financial constraints, including lack of health insurance, as well as language and cultural barriers to care. Increasing diversity of providers is an important step.

Locating services in accessible sites, such as schools and churches, can increase utilization. It is important to provide basic reproductive information, including information about fetal development and prenatal medical health. Professionals additionally need to be aware of the increased danger of preterm birth (especially in younger teens), low birth weight, and newborn mortality [32].

School-Based Services

These programs provide support, parenting education, child care, and other services for teen parents through their school. The first school-based clinics opened in the 1970s. In 1986, the Robert Wood Johnson Foundation established the School-based

Adolescent Health Care Program, spurring the formation of multiple school-based clinics (https://www.ncbi.nlm.nih.gov/books/NBK232693/), which have continued to evolve since then. These programs provide comprehensive health care to adolescents, with reproductive health services included as an important component.

School-based programs make sense in terms of easy access and help with encouragement to complete high school. Modern-day school-based programs vary. Some are strictly based in school; others include home visiting programs. Some schools include childcare at the schools themselves. This model seems to be especially helpful in that it not only provides day care, but also provides an opportunity for staff to model good child care for young parents. In addition, not only do in-school childcare services allow adolescent parents to continue/complete school, knowing their children are cared for, but they can also provide respite for family caregivers during regular hours of school [35].

In 1972 in the USA, Title IX of the Education Amendments was passed, making student pregnancy and parenthood the responsibility of any school that was federally funded. Quite forward thinking, this law prohibited expulsion of pregnant and parenting students and also promoted the development of school programs that would encourage students to complete high school and prevent repeat pregnancies [39]. These eventually evolved into two basic types of programs: "free-standing programs" that offered general education and parenting curriculum separate from mainstream classes and "supplemental programs" that offered parenting electives in continued mainstream schooling [39].

School-based programs have been shown to have many benefits. They have a positive effect on the educational success of pregnant and parenting teens, by reducing rates of absenteeism and dropout and increasing rates of high school graduation [36]. The component of parenting education has been shown to improve maternal interactions with their infants with regard to responsiveness, affective availability, and directiveness [26]. Infants of teen mothers who receive these services have fewer developmental delays and more positive interactions with their mothers. They respond more positively to physical contact and have greater affective stability [40].

The following are some examples of school-based programs with measurable outcomes.

Celotto Child Care Center This center was located within an urban high school in New Haven, Connecticut, and enrolled 52 adolescents 14–19 years old and their children from 1995 to 1998. Parents enrolled in the program were required to attend school/classes regularly, including a daily parent education class. Students also had to spend at least an hour per week in the childcare center and engage in parenting skills workshops with the day care providers. Students either paid for day care themselves or via public assistance funds for which they applied. This particular program also included home visiting services for those students encountering barriers to remaining in school, including difficulty with transportation or housing or legal problems [43].

Outcomes studied were school completion/continuation, grade point averages (GPAs), repeat birth rates, and child physical examination status and immunization rates. Results showed that the parent absence rate was 32%. Their mean grade point average (GPA) went from 1.74 pre-enrollment to 2.3. There was a correlation between rates of school attendance and GPAs. There were no repeat births, and 100% of those who continued enrollment at the childcare center through the duration of the study completed high school. Finally, 94% of the children who were enrolled at the child care center through the entire study period were current with their physical examinations, and 90% had up to date immunization rates.

From this study came a descriptive cross-sectional pilot study, in which formal measures of parent self-esteem (including confidence and competence), parenting stress, quality of parent–child interaction, and child development were used [35]. This study demonstrated high scores for maternal confidence with low scores for parenting stress. Parent–child interactions were also found to be of higher quality when compared to those results of an age-matched group on parenting adolescents and their children taken from a national database. In this study, 77% of the children of parenting adolescents were found to be "within normal limits" for the five subdomains measured: perceptual-fine motor, cognitive, language, gross motor, and self-care (such as holding a cup). This study overall found positive impact of this particular school-based system on parental competence and parent–child interactions.

Chelsea High School Program The Chelsea High School Program in Massachusetts, established in 2011, provides academic assistance and physical and mental health services for pregnant and parenting adolescents. The program is part of the Massachusetts Pregnant and Parenting Teen Initiative (MPPTI), in five communities throughout Massachusetts. Data from the program indicates that from 2014-2016, MPPTI served over 1,150 participants (570 adolescents and more than 600 children) in Chelsea, Holyoke, Lawrence, New Bedford, and Springfield. Among participants who were engaged in the program for 6 months or more:

- The percent of participants with full-time employment doubled.
- 98% were enrolled in health insurance.
- 93% reported using any contraception method.
- 58% made progress toward individualized academic and/or career goals.

The program in Chelsea, a city near Boston with a large Hispanic immigrant population, is conceptualized with three main "arms": academics, physical health, and mental health. Assistance with academics is provided by the outreach worker/liaison. Physical health is attended to by a school nurse practitioner, who is an employee of Massachusetts General Hospital (MGH). Mental health is provided offsite, usually within a few weeks of referral, at a local MGH site; patients are often referred by the nurse practitioner (personal communication, Ms. Jordan Hampton, September 2017).

The ninth grade outreach worker/expectant and parenting liaison is central to this program in her two-fold role. In her outreach role, she becomes familiar with many of the ninth graders. Because she is present from the beginning of high school, students may feel more comfortable talking to her about life, relationships, and challenges; she also astutely observes their behaviors and the relationships that they develop. In addition, she provides academic support in this role. In the expectant and parenting liaison role, her job is to provide supports and resources once a student lets her know that she is pregnant and the pregnancy is confirmed, or once a pregnant student is referred to her. At this point, the liaison will complete the intake, gathering information on due date, father of the child, in-home supports, prenatal care, financial assistance, and so on. She makes a checklist of where help is necessary. After the intake, the student is seen on an as-needed basis, and the liaison does more "behind-the-scenes" work, including connecting them to resources both in the school and in the community, as well as regularly auditing grades to make sure no failing grades are given if the assignments themselves were never given to the student to complete (personal communication with Ms. Elizabeth Portnoy, outreach worker/expecting and parenting student liaison at Chelsea High School, September 2017).

From 2012 to 2017, the Chelsea high school program worked with 122 expectant and parenting students, 35 of whom earned a diploma (22 were still active as students; 9 earned a certificate of attainment (finished class requirements but were not able to pass the standardized test to graduate); 41 dropped out; 1 was incarcerated; the others transferred to a different city or state). Almost 100% received prenatal care. There was one repeat pregnancy, but the majority of adolescents who gave birth received long acting reversable contraception after the first pregnancy.

Support for Pregnant and Parenting Teens Another example of a successful school-based program is Connecticut's Supports for Pregnant and Parenting Teens (SPPT), which was implemented in school districts with the highest rates of teen pregnancy and school dropouts. This program was funded by a grant from the Pregnancy Assistance Fund Resource of the USA Office of Adolescent Health. Providers on the team include a social worker, a part-time nurse, the local advisory committee, and other staff as necessary (such as a fatherhood coordinator). Their coordinated model helped to offer flexible yet quality schooling to students, case management and family support, referrals to necessary prenatal care and reproductive health services, links to child care, and education on parenting and basic life skills. Outcomes examined were reduction in second pregnancies, as well as graduation from high school (personal communication with Mr. Gerald Barrett, Grants Coordinator for the Institute of Teaching and Learning of the Capital Region Education Council, in February 2016 and September 2017, and website, which has since been taken down).

Most recent data from April 2017 showed a total of 187 students enrolled in the program, with 71 expectant mothers, 73 mothers, 24 expectant fathers, and 19 fathers. School attendance was an average of 75%. The services that were utilized the most were: parenting skills (97% of adolescents used this), concrete supports (95%), healthy relationships (94%), case management (93%), academic supports (78%), vocational services (66%), home visiting (64%), health care services (63%), child care (50%), and transportation (42%). In the 2015–2016 school year, 66% of students advanced to the next grade level and 82% of seniors graduated. 9% had repeat pregnancies. The program strove to involve teen fathers as well and included a "fatherhood coordinator" on staff (this program was in its nascent stages when the program lost funding). In addition, counselors were sent to these schools in order to educate teachers and staff about teen pregnancy and parenting to help decrease stigma of being a pregnant teen or teen mother. Sharing these and other such resources with this population of teens and helping to decrease stigma is clearly valuable (personal communication with Mr. Gerald Barrett).

The Office of Adolescent Health named the SPPT a "model program" and credited it with creating a "roadmap" of services for pregnant and parenting adolescents and helping them to complete their high school educations. However, due to the change in federal administration and recent focuses on more abstinence-based programs, this program is no longer in existence as of 2017 (personal communication with Mr. Gerald Barrett).

In summary, school-based programs offer a multidisciplinary approach, with the dual aims of enabling adolescent parents to complete school and be competent parents. They often provide on-site child care, medical services for both mothers and children, pregnancy, and parenting education. Prevention of future pregnancies during adolescence is also a goal.

Home Visiting Programs

Home visitors work with adolescent parents and their children in their own homes. This addresses the barrier of transportation to obtaining care and services. It also allows providers to see parents interacting with their children in their natural settings, as well as assess for other home issues that can be addressed. The home visitor works to form a therapeutic bond with the parent and model appropriate ways of interacting with the child, including setting limits [15].

The roots of these programs date as far back as the 1500s in Elizabethan England (http://homevisiting.org/history/timeline#0). Home-based services in the USA were described in the literature as early as the 1970s [15]. These services have continued to evolve over time to the evidence-based programs described here. They offer education, emotional supports, and other concrete supports [5]. In addition, many programs hope to create linkages to community resources and ongoing healthcare [27].

In 2010, evidence-based home visiting was "scaled up" with the federal Maternal, Infant and Early Childhood Home Visiting Program (MIECHV), which was part of the Affordable Care Act, and is jointly administered by the Health Resources and Services Administration (HRSA) and the Administration for Children and Families. It was then reauthorized under the Medicare Access and CHIP Reauthorization Act in 2015. This act mandated that any federally funded home visiting services had to serve "high-need" communities. The MIECHV has given grants totaling $1.9 million to states in order to broaden home visiting programs across the US and to support research of these programs [27]. Per the MIECHV website, as of fiscal year 2017, 18 programs met criteria for "evidence-based effectiveness" (https://mchb.hrsa.gov/sites/default/files/mchb/Maternal ChildHealthInitiatives/HomeVisiting/pdf/programbrief.pdf). Of newly enrolled households in fiscal year 2017, 22% included pregnant adolescents. Some of these evidence-based programs are described below.

Nurse-Family Partnership The Nurse-Family Partnership (NFP; www.nursefamilypartnership.org), the best studied program, was first developed in the 1970s by David Olds, PhD, and has shown continued improvement in keeping children of young, low income, first-time mothers safe and healthy and bettering the lives of young mothers and their children. The program serves low-income, unmarried, adolescent women [30]. The decision to focus on first-time mothers was based on the assumption that they would be more receptive to home visiting help and that the impact would be the greatest, as the home visiting nurses would then help with further family planning, as well as improve parenting skills for further children [30]. The home visiting program begins in pregnancy and continues until the child turns 2 years old. The goals are:

1. improving pregnancy outcomes (improving prenatal health),
2. improving child health and development, namely by improving parent understanding and sensitivity toward their child, as well as improving parental competency,
3. improving life course of parents, namely by assisting them with better family planning, finishing school, and finding jobs [30].

Home visiting nurses have formal training in women's and children's health. Home visits last 60–75 min. During these visits, nurses follow specific guidelines designed to address challenges at specific points during pregnancy and the first 2 years of a child's life [30]. Visiting nurses focus on targeting specific behaviors that would impact pregnancy outcomes, child development, and future life course for the mother; building strong relationships with supportive family and friends; and creating linkages with health and other services in the community. Nurses also seek to improve parent–child interactions after the child is born, and help mothers set goals and problem-solve on possible barriers to completing school and/or finding a job.

Three randomized controlled trials have been conducted—in Elmira, New York; Memphis, Tennessee; and Denver, Colorado. Results have consistently shown improved care of the child by the parent, as reflected by fewer injuries and ingestions, as well as improved emotional and language development in infants. In addition, the NFP has also shown improvement in life course of the mother, as indicated by reductions in repeat pregnancies, higher levels of employment, and decreased dependence on welfare services [30].

The NFP annual report for 2020 indicated over 58,323 families were served throughout the USA with over 1.8 million total visits (during 2020 92% of visits were by telehealth). This program is special in that it formed its own nonprofit organization, the NFP National Service Office (NSO), to ensure that replications of the NFP all had high fidelity and that nurses were well-educated and consistent in delivery of home visiting services. In addition, the NSO also used a uniform web-based system to monitor the quality of services delivered and improve implementation and expansion. Randomized controlled trials were conducted prior to opening the NFP program to public investment in new communities. In addition, results from these trials helped in the foundation of the evidence base for MIECHV [31]. The NSO continues to study and improve the guidelines and interventions of the NFP.

Healthy Families Massachusetts This program is an affiliate of Healthy Families America (HFA), which was started in 1992 by Prevent Child Abuse America. The goal of this home visiting initiative was to decrease rates of child abuse in children 5 years old and younger (http://www.healthyfamiliesamerica.org/site-finder /site-finder). On their website, one can find references for different randomized controlled studies in eight states. Per the website, Health Families programs are in 35 states and Washington, DC, Canada, and 6 US territories and together serve 100,000 families every year (http://www.healthyfamiliesamerica.org/state-evaluations/).

HFM (http://healthyfamiliesma.org/) is the only universal statewide home visiting program that targets and serves first-time young parents [17]. In a randomized controlled trial that assigned 704 participants to home visiting services (433 participants) or to a control group "referral and information only" (271 participants), outcomes were obtained at 12 and 24 months after initial enrollment. The control group received referral and information only. Eligibility applied to first-time parents who were less than 21 years old, and enrollment could occur from pregnancy up to the child's first birthday. Services continued through the child's third birthday. Goals of this program were to:

1. Prevent child abuse/neglect by bolstering effective parenting skills.
2. Support the child's health and development.
3. Promote educational achievement and improve job and life skills.
4. Prevent the occurrence of repeat pregnancies while still in adolescence.
5. Support the parent's physical and mental health [17].

Home visitors were paraprofessionals, some of them past recipients (or "graduates") of HFM home visiting services themselves. Home visitors received several hours of training and had multiple supervision sessions for each client to which they were assigned. Although there was a general curriculum to be followed, teaching was tailored to the needs of the clients in a non-stigmatizing or shaming way (personal communication with Ms. Sarita Rogers, Director of Home Visiting at The Children's Trust, in July 2017). The goal was biweekly visits for prenatal participants, weekly visits after the birth of the child through 6 months (or 6 months after enrollment for those participants who enrolled after the birth of the child). On average, mothers had 24 home visits over 14.7 months, which was fewer than intended by HFM. Almost 14% of women in the home visiting arm did not receive home visiting services at all [17].

Positive effects included that first-time mothers learned better control of stress, engaged in fewer risky behaviors (decreased drug use, decreased partner violence, increased condom use), and made educational attainment. Home visiting services also had a statistically significant impact upon college attendance by young mothers [17]. When followed out 60 and 72 months post-enrollment, more subtle differences were found, as "subgroups" were also examined: young mothers with depression, with history of childhood maltreatment, and with low or high family supports (http://ase.tufts.edu/tier/documents/tuftsFinalReportExecutiveSummary2017.pdf). They also evaluated "dosage effects" of number of home visits on outcomes.

The group found no overall program effects on supporting effective parenting when examining rates of maltreatment, reports of parenting stress, parental discipline of their children, and observed mother–child interactions. For subgroups of mothers with lower family support upon enrollment, mothers receiving home visiting services reported less parental stress when their children were preschool age than the control group. In addition, mothers who were more depressed at enrollment reported less corporal punishment of their children. With regard to promoting child development, an improvement in working memory in preschool children was noted in the home visiting services group versus the control group. There were no differences in outcomes for child readiness for school or emotion regulation. More promising outcomes were that mothers were less likely to report homelessness (28% for home visiting services vs 41% for control group), and mothers who did not report depressive symptoms at time of enrollment were more likely to have graduated from college. Mothers who had more home visits were less likely to have repeat pregnancies. Fewer depressive symptoms were reported by mothers in the preschool period, and there was decreased substance abuse among mothers in the kindergarten period. In addition to the five goals mentioned above, this study added another goal: encouraging advocacy and utilization of early childhood systems of care. For this goal, it was found that there were fewer Emergency Department visits and that mothers were more likely to advocate for their child's needs rather than to be passive. In addition, mothers with fewer family supports were found to have better relationships with their children's teachers or childcare providers during the kindergarten period [9].

Parents as Teachers (PAT; https://parentsasteachers.org/) The PAT program is another evidence-based home visiting program. It began in 1981 in Missouri [42]. This program promotes healthy development of children prenatally through 5 years old via support of the parents by home visitors. The four core components of the PAT model are: personal visits (two times a month to once a month, depending on needs of the family), group connections (monthly), child screenings, and resource network. The home visitors, or "parent educators" receive intensive training in a specific curriculum with which to work with the families they serve, and receive ongoing support and supervision for their caseloads.

This program has been demonstrated in randomized controlled studies to improve parenting skills and reduce child maltreatment [3, 18] and improve school readiness, school behavior, and academic performance [21]. Additional benefits include early detection of developmental delays, and adherence to recommended immunization schedules.

In summary, home visiting programs have the advantage of delivering care in the most accessible way possible, the adolescent's home. The home visitor is able to interact with others in the home as well as the young mother, and can support co-parenting by family members. These programs can also serve adolescents who are not in school. There are some questions about the overall effects of these programs and whether they are cost effective, as outcomes have been mixed. The experience of the Healthy Families Massachusetts program suggests that particular subgroups of adolescents – those who are depressed or lack family support, for example, might benefit the most.

Community Outreach Programs

Community outreach can be defined as a collaborative approach between a service organization and an at risk population; community outreach workers are usually drawn from the communities they serve, but can also be health care workers affiliated with a clinic or hospital. The aim is to link vulnerable individuals with the health care and social services they need. One of the hallmarks of community outreach is that it is mobile; that is, workers are out in the community instead of based in an office [38]. Community outreach programs can focus on a variety of needs that are not met by traditional services, for example, breast cancer screenings in low-income communities. A number of outreach programs are aimed at helping young parents. A few examples are described below.

The **Young Parents' Outreach Center (YPOC)** is a program located in St. Mary's Home, a not-for-profit charitable organization for young parents in Ottawa, Canada, that provides services for pregnant and parenting youth up to 18 years of age and their children, including emergency shelter, continuing education, medical clinics, cooking classes, pregnancy groups, playgroups, and counseling [13].

This multidisciplinary program provides a full range of health-related services, including mental health services for young pregnant women, fathers, and infants. The medical component is staffed by a nurse and pediatrician, and has community partnerships with family medicine, obstetrics, and psychiatry. The focus of the program is on supporting parenting self-confidence and self-esteem; providing medical care and anticipatory guidance regarding child developmental stages and adolescent developmental stages, and offering other medical care such as birth-control counseling and mental health care. Mental health concerns were the primary reason pregnant and parenting young people were referred to this program; the program reported fewer missed appointments compared with hospital-based mental health clinics [28].

The **Young Mother's Project of ROCA, Inc.** (https://rocainc.org/) is a program in Chelsea and other communities in Massachusetts. Its target population is young mothers (16–24 years old) who have one or more of the following risk factors: being single, gang- and street-involved, engaged in substance abuse, involved in the justice system, have a history of violence and trauma, have dropped out of high school, and have no employment history. Referrals are from hospitals, schools, police, home visiting services, and probation officers and often consist only of names and addresses. Five to six youth workers, ranging in age from the 20s to 50s, are assigned about 25 mothers each to work with. The first 4–6 months consists of what the program directors term "relentless outreach." In this model, the youth workers find the young mothers in the community and continuously reach out, trying to build an alliance, even as they are being turned away. On average, it takes this long to eventually bring the young mother into services. Outreach then occurs about twice a week (personal communication with Mr. Yotam Zeira, July 2017).

The program is a 4-year "adapted dual generation model," which is "intensive mother-focused intervention with child elements." This consists of 2 years of intensive programming and relationship building followed by 2 years of follow-up and support to sustain change. Services offered include support of education/GED preparation, transitional employment (mothers must work 60 consecutive work-days before they can obtain recommendations to work in the community), life skills, parenting skills, cognitive-behavioral therapy delivered by paraprofessionals using a curriculum developed with Massachusetts General Hospital, community building ("Wednesday Family Night," during which these mothers take classes and have dinners with other young mothers in the program, while their children are provided with daycare), dual programming for mother and child, and less intensive child services (child care with light early education, developmental and social emotional assessments, referral to early intervention as necessary).

Fiscal year 2020 results demonstrated successful outreach to 254 high-risk young mothers and 335 young children, with 80% retention in the program. Of these, 88% engaged in programming training, 89% had delayed subsequent pregnancies, 33 young mothers enrolled in the transitional employment program, and 43 young mothers were placed at a job in the community (with 74% keeping these jobs for at least 3 months (https://rocainc.org/how-we-do-it/outcomes/young-mothers/).

Medical Home Programs or Programs Embedded in Primary Care Clinics

The term medical home refers to a model of delivery of primary care in an efficient, "one stop shopping" model. Primary care, along with case management, social work, and mental health concerns are all assessed and addressed in some capacity, either directly in the clinic, or via referrals to community services [15].

This model is also known as Patient or Family Centered Medical Home; a precursor to the medical home, the so-called Teen-tot programs, was first described in the 1980s. Most of the care is provided within the practice, with referrals outside as needed. The medical home includes a multidisciplinary team, which is responsible for coordinating care and making sure that all of the patient's health care needs are met. The practice engages in quality improvement. This model is well suited to young parents and their children, who would normally have to get care in separate settings. These programs make both medical care and psychosocial supports available to both adolescent parents and their children in an easily accessible manner. The American Academy of Pediatrics has endorsed the medical home model for young parents, citing extensive evidence documenting improvements in quality and efficiency with this approach.

Project Raising Adolescent Families Together is one such program, [6]. This program in Massachusetts enrolled adolescent parents within a week of delivery. An evaluation of the program found high rates of child immunization (above national, state, and local benchmarks); higher than national average rates of well-visits for publicly insured children (both for children and adolescents); significantly increased use of condoms over the 2-year follow-up; and almost 50% of adolescent mothers using a depot contraception method. The rate of repeat pregnancy was 14.7% at 1 year follow-up and 24.6% at 2 year follow-up, which was lower than the 42% at 2 year follow-up in other reports [6]. As use of depot injections is associated with lower rates of repeat pregnancy, the higher percentage of adolescents who used this method may account for the lower levels of repeat pregnancies in this population. In addition, a 1-year follow-up demonstrated fewer depressive symptoms, correlated with an increase in supports [2]. Longitudinal results also showed higher school continuation rates (77.6% at 1 year and 68.7% at 2 years) and higher rates of employment for parenting adolescents than rates for all adolescents in Massachusetts. At 24 months follow-up, the majority of adolescent mothers were living independently; 36.8% remained living with their parents or other family members [6].

Mom Power Program Another program, the Mom Power Program at the University of Michigan, sought to pair mental health and parenting services in a community primary care setting [22]. Through a multimodal, multi-collaborative Corner Clinic Teen Parent Program, adolescent mothers and their children received services including primary and obstetric care, mental health care, counseling (parenting, couples, group), and referrals to other social support programs [22]. The Mom Power parenting group was one of the forms of counseling offered, consisting of a curriculum covering psychoeducational parenting skills, as well as skills for self-care. In the group setting, providers were also able to observe the children of adolescent mothers and offer screening for developmental days and emotion regulation. The target population was mothers 15–21 years old and their children 0–6 years old. The duration of the group was for 10 weeks, and it focused on improving mother–child interactions, strengthening parenting skills, managing self-care, establishing relationships within the healthcare system, and building social support structure. Preliminary results from the Mom Power Group on 23 adolescent mothers (average age 19.6 years) showed an average of 1–2 children each (average age 16 months), mostly single, predominantly minority in ethnicity, the majority with less than high school education, and predominantly of low income. They had all experienced an average of five traumatic life events; half met criteria for post-traumatic stress disorder (PTSD), and half met criteria for major depressive disorder (MDD). During the course of the Mom Power Group, adolescent mothers experienced an average of an additional two traumatic events. However, by the end of the program, only one (down from 10) participant continued to meet criteria for PTSD, and seven (down from 13) still met criteria for major depressive disorder. Adolescent mothers also rated themselves as "less guilty and ashamed" about their parenting skills when comparing pre- vs. post-group assessment.

Co-parenting Groups

Supporting parenting competence, which includes both parenting self-efficacy and satisfaction, can improve how parents care for and raise their children and also improve child health outcomes [1]. Social supports, including family and friends, can increase parenting competence, but adolescent parents often have lower levels of peer supports than adolescents who are not parents [7]. In a study of 231 young couples, with women aged 14–21 years and in their 2nd or 3rd trimester of pregnancy and men age 14 years or older, results demonstrated that a strong support structure and healthy family functioning bolstered parenting competence in both young mother and fathers [1]. In addition, research has shown that support of the baby's father also has a beneficial effect on the mother's sense of parenting competence [34]. A strong co-parenting relationship is the best predictor for positive involvement of the father. In addition, positive co-parenting has a direct and positive effect on child behavioral outcomes [19].

Two examples of co-parenting groups are The Young Parenthood Program and Strong Foundations. Both groups help to build skills for better communication and conflict management, as well as self-regulation [15]. Both programs focus on bolstering co-parenting skills.

The Young Parenthood Program The Young Parenthood Program consists of a 10-week counseling program that occurs during pregnancy [11]. The main focus of this intervention is on supporting interpersonal relationships between pregnant adolescent mothers and their partners, with the goal of improving the parents' relationship and parenting of their child. To study the effectiveness of this program, 105 pregnant adolescents and their partners were divided into the Young Parenthood Program group or treatment as usual. Mothers had to be primiparous, be between 14 and 18 years old, be less than 26 weeks pregnant, and have a willing partner in the intervention (biological father). Co-parenting skills and parent functioning were assessed during the second trimester, 12 weeks post-partum, and 18 months post-partum [11].

The Young Parenthood Program is divided into five phases. The first phase works on building therapeutic alliance and helps young parents-to-be to understand the relationship between co-parenting and child development. The second phase helps to establish relationship goals and which interpersonal skills are necessary to achieve those goals. The third phase employs activities meant to build communication and self-regulation skills that correlate with positive parenting. The fourth phase concentrates on navigating the transition to parenthood. The final phase examines future co-parenting issues, such as family planning (and preventing repeat pregnancies) [11].

Results from this study demonstrated that young fathers had a higher likelihood of staying engaged in raising their children and reported having better relationships with their partners. In addition, the study found that many of the positive effects on fathers were mediated through the mother's improvement in relational competence. Positive parenting and co-parenting included more nurturing behavior from fathers and decreased child abuse potential scores. This study also found that YPP seemed to be more effective for fathers than their partners [11]. As adolescent parents are at high risk for interpersonal violence, YPP has great potential in terms of improving the home environment for the child.

Strong Foundations Strong Foundations is a program designed to enable and bolster co-parenting skills in adolescent couples. Unlike YPP, Strong Foundations consists of five prenatal group sessions and then nine individual post-partum sessions that are integrated into the child's well-visit checks in a teen-tot primary care program during the first year of life [23]. The intervention was adapted from Family Foundations, an adult co-parenting support program. The program targets low-income, urban, minority youth. The intervention focuses on teaching and then allowing young parents to practice (usually via role-play) communication, problem-solving, and relaxation skills. Preliminary results indicated the feasibility of the program and its acceptability in this population. Adolescent parents rated the information as helpful and likely to be used in the future. The authors noted the importance of recruiting young fathers directly, and found they were enthusiastic participants, contrary to prevalent assumptions that they would not be interested. Only 7% of fathers with eligible partners refused to participate.

General Interventions

Other general interventions in adolescent pregnancy and parenting that have some evidence for being helpful include scheduling social work visits during clinical appointment times, providing education in the waiting room, provider-initiated discussions on family planning, and reminder calls and letters for appointments [29]. Compared to a control group, those receiving these extra interventions have lower rates of high school dropout and repeat pregnancy; and higher rates of infant immunization [29]. Hodgkinson et al. [14] suggest that modifying this model by including mental health supports and treatment could improve overall care for this population even further.

Public Policy Initiatives

While most federally funded programs in the USA have focused primarily on pregnancy prevention, there have been some initiatives that have focused on supporting young parents. Through the Office of the Assistant Secretary for Health of the Department of Health and Human Services, competitive grants were provided from 2010 to 2019 to support both mothers and fathers through a program known as the Pregnancy Assistance Fund, funded by the US Patient Protection and Affordable Care Act of 2010 (https://opa.hhs.gov/grant-programs/pregnancy-assistance-fund-paf). This initiative had a particular focus on mental health, substance use, teen parenting, and engaging teen fathers. Under the program, funding was established that provided grants to states and tribes to improve the health, social, educational, and economic outcomes for expectant and parenting teens and young adults, their children, and their families. The program served close to 110,000 expectant and parenting teens, women, fathers, and their families, who received a wide range of support services related to personal health, child health, parenting, education, and employment, as well as concrete supports like diapers and baby equipment.

The goal of the Pregnancy Assistance Fund was to improve outcomes of pregnant and parenting adolescents and their families. Grants were administered to 27 states and 4 tribal entities. Special attention was paid to programs serving vulnerable populations, including male, Latino, Native American, and LGBTQ youth. Programs funded by this project aimed to support pregnant and parenting adolescents and their families in multiple settings (including schools and community service centers), prevent intimate partner violence and offer interventions, promote partnerships, and improve dissemination and sustainability of such services. A bill to reauthorize the program was introduced in 2019 and again in 2020 but as of this writing has not passed.

Discussion

Well-designed programs for young parents can help to reduce the negative effects of stigma and social adversity. Organized services and programs can help pregnant and parenting adolescents to move toward self-sufficiency, while also balancing the demands of parenting. They can bolster existing supports, offer additional supports, decrease stigma, and empower young parents to ask for further services for their children and for themselves. In doing so, these services support developing healthy family structures, strengthen communities, and demonstrate respect for adolescent rights and their capacity to succeed.

As noted above, outcome data showing efficacy are available for individual programs. In addition, a systematic review published in 2020 of programs for teenage parents and their children found evidence for efficacy of a variety of approaches, although also noting the limitations of much of the research [12].

Many of the programs described in this chapter are supported by or were originally supported by federal grants. Other programs are supported by public donations or institutions themselves (such as the Chelsea High School Program, which was initially supported by funds from the Office of Adolescent Health). As always with grant-funded programs, sustainability is an issue. Funding is subject to the prioritization of such programs by federal agencies, elected officials, and the general public. Demonstration of efficacy is crucial but may not be sufficient. Ultimately, local public support is essential to continue funding. Programs tended to have the most impact on aspects that they identified as their goals, for example contraceptive use following pregnancy. One size does not fit all; various approaches can work; and programs need to be tailored to fit the needs of the teens they serve. Challenges are hiring and training of personnel, adapting programs to special populations, and recruitment of teens, especially teen fathers.

As a society, we cannot become complacent with the knowledge that adolescent pregnancy is declining. There should be continued advocacy for pregnancy prevention and encouragement of safe sexual practices, including medically accurate sexual education and use of contraception. Supporting programs to help adolescent mothers with family planning, including using contraception and avoiding repeat pregnancies during adolescence, could therefore be beneficial to adolescent mothers and society as a whole. In addition to prevention efforts, there should be more emphasis on helping pregnant and parenting adolescents to become better equipped to be responsive and understanding parents and encourage them to achieve higher education and employment. Programs such as the school-based services, home visiting services, community outreach programs, embedded medical model services, and co-parenting groups highlighted in this chapter seek to increase opportunities for pregnant youth and young parents and their children, and to empower them to make healthy decisions about parenting and life in order to procure a better future for their families.

References

1. Angley M, Divney A, Magriples U, Kershaw T. Social support, family functioning and parenting competence in adolescent parents. Matern Child Health J. 2015;19(1):67–73.
2. Brown JD, Harris SK, Woods ER, Buman MP, Cox JE. Longitudinal study of depressive symptoms and social support in adolescent mothers. Matern Child Health J. 2012;16(4):894–901.
3. Chaiyachati B, Gaither J, Hughes M, Foley-Schain K, Leventhal J. Preventing child maltreatment: examination of an established statewide home visiting program. J Child Abuse Negl. 2018;49:476–84.
4. Clarke J. It's not all doom and gloom for teenage mothers – exploring the factors that contribute to positive outcomes. Int J Adolesc Youth. 2015;20(4):470–84.
5. Council on Child and Adolescent Health American Academy of Pediatrics. The role of home-visitation programs in improving health outcomes for children and families. Pediatrics. 1998;101(3):486–9.

6. Cox JE, Buman M, Woods ER, Famakinwa O, Harris SK. Evaluation of raising adolescent families together program: a medical home for adolescent mothers and their children. Am J Public Health. 2012;102(10):1879–85.
7. Crase SJ, Hockaday C, Cooper McCarville P. Brief report: perceptions of positive and negative support: do they differ for pregnant/parenting adolescents and non-pregnant, non-parenting adolescents? J Adolesc. 2007;30(3):505–12.
8. Decker MJ, Pineda N, Gutmann-Gonzalez A, Brindis CD. Youth-centered maternity care: a binational qualitative comparison of the experiences and perspectives of Latina adolescents and healthcare providers. BMC Pregnancy Childbirth. 2021;21(1):349. https://doi.org/10.1186/s12884-021-03831-4.
9. Easterbrooks A, Chaudhuri J, Fauth R, Contreras M Kotake C, Moosmann D. The Massachusetts healthy families Evaluation-2: early childhood (MHFE-2EC): follow-up study of a randomized, controlled trial of a statewide home visiting program for young parents. Medford, Massachusetts: Tufts Interdisciplinary Evaluation Research (TIER) Eliot-Pearson Department of Child Study and Human Development Department of Urban and Environmental Policy and Planning, Tufts University; 2017.
10. Fleming N, O'Driscoll T, Becker G, Spitzer RF. Adolescent pregnancy guidelines. J Obstet Gynaecol Can: JOGC (Journal d'obstetrique et Gynecologie Du Canada: JOGC). 2015;37(8):740–56. https://doi.org/10.1016/S1701-2163(15)30180-8.
11. Florsheim P, Burrow-Sanchez JJ, Minami T, McArthur L, Heavin S, Hudak C. Young parenthood program: supporting positive paternal engagement through coparenting counseling. Am J Public Health. 2012;102(10):1886–92.
12. Harding JF, Knab J, Zief S, Kelly K, McCallum D. A systematic review of programs to promote aspects of teen parents' self-sufficiency: supporting educational outcomes and healthy birth spacing. Matern Child Health J. 2020;24(Suppl 2):84–104. https://doi.org/10.1007/s10995-019-02854-w.
13. Harrison ME, Weinstangel H, Dalziel N, Moreau KA. A collaborative outreach clinic for pregnant youth and adolescent mothers: description of a pilot clinic and its patients. Paediatr Child Health. 2014;19(5):247–50. https://doi.org/10.1093/pch/19.5.247.
14. Hodgkinson SC, Colantuoni E, Roberts D, Berg-Cross L, Belcher HM. Depressive symptoms and birth outcomes among pregnant teenagers. J Pediatr Adolesc Gynecol. 2010;23(1):16–22.
15. Hodgkinson S, Beers L, Southammakosane C, Lewin A. Addressing the mental health needs of pregnant and parenting adolescents. Pediatrics. 2014;133:114–22.
16. Hofferth SL, Reid L, Mott FL. The effects of early childbearing on schooling over time. Fam Plan Perspect. 2011;33(6):259–67.
17. Jacobs F, Easterbrooks A, Goldberg J, Mistry J, Bumgarner E, Raskin M, Foss N, Fauth R. Improving adolescent parenting: results from a randomized controlled trial of a home visiting program for young families. Am J Public Health. 2016;106:342–9.
18. Jonson-Reid M, Drake B, Constantino J, Tandom M, Pons L, Kohl P, Roesch S, Wideman E, Dunnigan A, Auslander W. A randomized trial of home visitation for CPS-involved families: the moderating impact of maternal depression and CPS history. Child Maltreat. 2018;23:281–93. *
19. Karreman A, van Tuijl C, van Aken MA, Dekovic M. Parenting, coparenting, and effortful control in preschoolers. J Fam Psychol. 2008;22(1):30–40.
20. Lachance CR, Burrus BB, Scott AR. Building an evidence base to inform interventions for pregnant and parenting adolescents: a call for rigorous evaluation. Am J Public Health. 2012;102:1826–32.
21. Lahti M, Evans CBR, Goodman G, Cranwell Schmidt M, LeCroy CW. Parents as teachers (PAT) home-visiting intervention: a path to improved academic outcomes, school behavior, and parenting skills. Child Youth Serv Rev. 2019;99:451–60.
22. LePlatte D, Rosenblum KR, Stanton E, Miller N, Muzik M. Mental health in primary care for adolescent parents. Ment Health Fam Med. 2012;9:39–45.

23. Lewin A, Hodgkinson S, Waters DM, Prempeh HA, Beers LS, Feinberg ME. Strengthening positive coparenting in teen parents: a cultural adaptation of an evidence-based intervention. J Prim Prev. 2015;36:139–54.
24. Martin JA, Hamilton BE, Osterman MJK, Driscoll AK. National vital statistics reports, vol. 70, no. 2, March 23, 2021. Atlanta, GA: Centers for Disease Control Division of Vital Statistics;2021. https://www.cdc.gov/nchs/data/nvsr/nvsr70/nvsr70-02-508.pdf
25. Maslowsky J, Powers D, Hendrick CE, Al-Hamoodah L. County-level clustering and characteristics of repeat vs first teen births in the United States, 2015–2017. J Adolesc Health. 2019;65(5):674–680.
26. Mayers H, Hager M, Buckner E. The chances for children teen parent-infant project: results of a pilot intervention for teen mothers and their infants in inner city high schools. Infant Ment Health J. 2008;29:320–42.
27. Minkovitz CS, O'Neill KMG, Duggan AK. Home visiting: a service strategy to reduce poverty and mitigate its consequences. Acad Pediatr. 2016;16:S105–11.
28. Norris S, Norris ML, Sibbald E, Aubry T, Harrison ME, Lafontaine G, Gandhi J. Demographic characteristics associated with pregnant and post-partum youth referred for mental health services in a community outreach center. J Can Acad Child Adolesc Psychiatry (Journal de l'Academie Canadienne de Psychiatrie de l'enfant et de l'adolescent). 2016;25(3):152–8.
29. O'Sullivan AL, Jacobsen BS. A randomized trial of a health care program for first-time adolescent mothers and their infants. Nurs Res. 1992;41(4):210–5.
30. Olds DL. The nurse-family partnership: an evidence-based preventive intervention. Infant Ment Health J. 2006;27(1):5–25.
31. Olds D, Donelan-McCall N, O'Brien R, MacMillan H, Jack S, Jenkins T, Dunlap WP, O'Fallon M, Yost E, Thorland B, Pinto F, Gasbarro M, Baca P, Melnick A, Beeber L. Improving the nurse-family partnership in community practice. Pediatrics. 2013;132:S110–7.
32. Powers ME, Takagishi J, Committee on Adolescence, Council on Early Childhood. Care of adolescent Parents and their children. Pediatrics. 2021;147(5):e2021050919.
33. Pinzon JL, Jones VF, Committee on Adolescence, & Committee on Early Childhood. Care of adolescent parents and their children. Pediatrics. 2012;130(6):e1743–56.
34. Roye CF, Balk SJ. The relationship of partner support to outcomes for teenage mothers and their children: a review. J Adolesc Health. 1996;19(2):86–93.
35. Sadler LS, Swartz MS, Ryan-Krause P. Supporting adolescent mothers and their children through a high school-based child care center and parent support program. J Pediatr Health Care. 2003;17:109–17.
36. Sadler L, Swartz M, Ryan-Krause P, Seitz V, Meadows-Oliver M, Grey M, Clemmens D. Promising outcomes in teen mothers enrolled in a school based parent support program and child care center. J Sch Health. 2007;77:121–30.
37. Seamark CJ, Lings P. Positive experiences of teenage motherhood: a qualitative study. Br J Gen Pract. 2004;54:813–8.
38. Shin HY, Kim KY, Kang P. Concept analysis of community health outreach. BMC Health Serv Res. 2020;20:417. https://doi.org/10.1186/s12913-020-05266-7.
39. Stevens-Simon C, Beach RK. School-based prenatal and postpartum care: strategies for meeting the medication and educational needs of pregnant and parenting students. J Sch Health. 1992;62(7):304–9.
40. Strunk J. The effect of school based health clinics on teenage pregnancy and parenting outcomes: an integrated literature review. J Sch Nurs. 2008;24:13–20.
41. Tilghman J, Lovette A. Prenatal care: the adolescent's perspective. J Perinat Educ. 2008;17(2):50–3. https://doi.org/10.1624/105812408X298390.
42. Wagner MM, Clayton SL. The parents as teachers program: results from two demonstrations. Futur Child. 1999;9(1):91–115.
43. Williams EG, Sadler LS. Effects of an urban high school-base child care center on self-selected adolescent parents and their children. J Sch Health. 2001;71(2):47–52.

Mental Health in Pregnant and Parenting Teens

8

Lois T. Flaherty

Psychiatric Illness as a Risk Factor for Teen Pregnancy

Psychiatric illness is, in addition to all of its many other negative consequences, a risk factor for teen pregnancy.

A US study two decades ago of a community sample (the National Comorbidity Survey, a nationally representative household survey) found a correlation between retrospectively reported early onset psychiatric disorders and subsequent teenage parenthood in the general population. [54]. This study used face-to-face interviews to collect the data from 5877 respondents aged 15–54 years. The data included DSM-III-R anxiety disorders, mood disorders, substance abuse disorders, and conduct disorder, age at the birth of the first child, and teenage sexual activity. Psychiatric disorders were found to be associated with teenage parenthood for both males and females, with significant odds ratios of 2.0–12.0. Disaggregation analyses showed that psychiatric disorders were associated with increased probability of sexual activity.

A later study that analyzed data from a large longitudinal study of adolescent health found depressive symptoms to be associated with earlier sexual debut, which might explain the link between depression and pregnancy [60]. Subsequently, Vigod and colleagues in Ontario, Canada, reported on a cross-sectional study using annual administrative health data on insurance claims for a large number of girls aged 15–19 years over several years (1999–2009) [102]. The total number of girls in the database each year of the study ranged from 379,303 to 437,534. Girls who had an index pregnancy were compared with those who did not with respect to their having had a major mental illness within 5 years of when they were estimated to have conceived (based on the date of birth). Major mental illness was defined as major depression, bipolar disorder or psychotic disorder. The overall rate of pregnancy

L. T. Flaherty (✉)
Harvard Medical School and Cambridge Health Alliance, Cambridge, MA, USA

J.-V. P. Wittenberg et al. (eds.), *Adolescent Pregnancy and Parenting*,
https://doi.org/10.1007/978-3-031-42502-8_8

among adolescents with pre-existing major mental illness was 44.9 per 1000 compared to 15.2 per 1000 unaffected girls; girls with major mental illness gave birth at three times the rate of those who did not have mental illness. The researchers further separated the girls with a history of primary psychotic disorder from those with a history of primary mood disorder. They found 29.3% of the births were to girls with a primary psychotic disorder and 70.6% were to girls with a primary mood disorder. Although they did find that multi-parity, low socioeconomic status, and living in a rural area independently increased the risk of teen births, these were not sufficient to explain the discrepancy as socio economic status or place of residence were similar in both groups. They also noted that fertility rates decreased over the 10 years of this study in both groups but less in the group with major mental illness. Rates of multiple births were also higher in the index group. The caveat to this study that it only measured live births, and thus was not a complete measure of pregnancy rates. The results do indicate that for a teenage girl, having a major mental illness is a risk factor for pregnancy. It is certainly likely that following the birth of a child to an adolescent with a major mental illness, both the mother and baby will be at further risk for adverse outcomes. Vigod and colleagues described children of adolescent mothers with mental illness as "doubly vulnerable" owing to having an adolescent parent and a parent with a major mental illness [102, p. e586].

Prevalence of Mental Health Problems

While there are few studies examining the mental health of pregnant teens, those we do have suggest the prevalence of mental health disorders is high. For example, a Brazilian study that looked at a low-income population of pregnant teenagers (aged 11 to 19) found about one third had at least one disorder [67]. However, as we saw in Chap. 1, the population of pregnant and parenting teens is largely drawn from a larger population who are living in conditions of psychosocial disadvantage because of poverty, minority status, family disruption and so on. Therefore, it becomes important to untangle the effects of adversity from the impact of pregnancy and childbearing.

Stefanie Mollborn, who has written extensively about teen pregnancy in the context of social disadvantage, and her colleague Elizabeth Morningstar, used data from two national surveys to assess "distress" among teen mothers [70]. They found "teenage mothers had higher levels of distress than their childless adolescent peers and adult mothers, but the experience of teenage child bearing did not appear to be the cause." Rather, pregnancy was more likely to occur among girls who were already distressed. Extreme psychological distress and extreme socioeconomic disadvantage were particularly predictive of teenage childbearing. The authors noted a number of problems with earlier work that found increased levels of depression in association with teen motherhood. The findings were based on smaller non-representative samples. There is also difficulty measuring depression pre-pregnancy if the studies are done retrospectively. Much of the data are artifactual as a result of the selection of distressed adolescents into motherhood. In contrast, they maintain that their findings indicate that being poor and distressed greatly increase the probability of childbearing, concluding "social disadvantage underlies both teenage childbearing and distress." Milan and colleagues [63]. compared "emotional distress" symptoms in pregnant (n = 203) and nulliparous adolescents (n = 188) from economically disadvantaged communities over an 18-month period. The prevalence of significant emotional distress was higher than adolescent norms for both groups but did not differ between the two groups. They did find a difference in how the symptoms developed over time. We will look at other studies that have attempted to separate pregnancy from psychosocial disadvantage in the sections on various disorders.

Psychosocial and Biological Aspects of Pregnancy and Their Influence on Mental Health

Multiple changes occur during and after pregnancy, including hormonal and psychosocial changes. Unlike what was commonly believed in the past, hormones and the state of being pregnant do not protect against mental illness.

Hormonal Changes Estrogen and progesterone quickly increase during the first trimester, plateau during the second and third trimesters, then rapidly drop postpartum. Both estrogen and progesterone mediate the serotonin system, the elevated levels of these hormones result in high serotonin levels in pregnancy followed by a rapid decrease postpartum, which can lead to significant mood changes. In addition, placental cortisol-releasing hormone (CRH) increases levels of cortisol, which affect the hypothalamic-pituitary axis (HPA), which may also increase the risk of depression.

Psychosocial Changes Psychosocially, the pregnant and postpartum woman must adjust in a change in role and balance coping with the pregnancy and baby with other areas of her life, balancing parenting with work, school, social, interpersonal, family, and other obligations. Rather than making choices only for herself, she must reframe her world using the mother–child dyad. For pregnant teenagers, this is exacerbated by their developmental stage, as they struggle to gain more autonomy from their parents and other authority figures, and as they explore their own identities. As we describe in the chapter on developmental trajectories, the young mother's adaptation to these demands will be influenced by many factors. These include the involvement of the father of the baby, the level of support or disapproval of her parents, and the level of acceptance in her community. For the pregnant adolescent struggling with psychiatric illness the stress and risk of adverse outcomes is compounded.

Depression

Depression has been the best studied condition during pregnancy and in the postpartum period.

Characteristics

Several types of depressive disorders are listed in the DSM-5 [4]. In addition to major depressive disorder, these include disruptive mood dysregulation disorder and dysthymia. Symptoms of depression include depressed mood or anhedonia for at least a 2-week period, accompanied by symptoms that include changes in sleep, appetite, energy, concentration, psychomotor activity, feelings of guilt or worthlessness, and/or suicidal ideation.

These disorders differ in terms of duration, timing, or presumed etiology, but all are characterized by sad, empty, or irritable mood. They all have in common mood and cognitive disturbances as well as somatic symptoms and impaired functioning.

Not included in this list is subclinical or subthreshold depression, a less well-defined condition in which severity of symptoms and impairment do not reach the level of a DSM diagnosis. The extant literature suggests that this form of depression is associated with significant distress and impairment [82], and neurobiological data support the argument that subthreshold depression is part of a continuum rather than a separate category [106].

Prevalence

Depression rates, low in childhood, begin to climb in early adolescence, around age 12, peaking at 16–17 years; the rate is consistently higher in girls than in boys. Depression affects a significant percentage of all teenagers, and epidemiological studies based on survey data show that rates of depression among adolescents and young adults have been increasing. The National Comorbidity Survey, conducted between 2001 and 2004, included over 10,000 adolescents between 13 and 18 years old. It found a lifetime prevalence of 11% for major depressive disorder and 12-month prevalence of 7.5% [10]. The rates were 2–3 times higher for female adolescents than for males and were highest in mid-late adolescence (the peak time for teen pregnancy).

Data from a large national annual survey conducted by the Substance Abuse and Mental Health Services Administration in the US (the National Surveys on Drug Use and Health; [69]) show the 12 month prevalence of major depressive episodes, which had stayed fairly constant during the first decade of the twenty-first century, went from 12% in 2010 to 17.3% in 2014 (in contrast, the rate for boys was 4.2% in 2010 and 5.7% in 2014). The survey also assessed contact with mental health services, which did not change over the years they studied, indicating that there was likely much more untreated depression. A breakdown of the data showed rates rising from 8 to 13.2% between 2009 and 2017 for both adolescents (12–17 years old) and young adults (18–25 years old). Rates were even higher—17.81%—for 16–17 year olds [98].

In Pregnant and Parenting Adolescents Depression is common during pregnancy and the postpartum period for women of all ages, including adolescents. The American College of Obstetrics and Gynecology reported that research shows approximately 14–23% of pregnant women experience depression during their pregnancy, and 5–25% experience depression postpartum (2015). Similar rates have been found in pregnant and parenting adolescents [97].

Coelho and colleagues in their study of low-income Brazilian adolescents found a prevalence of 13%. [22]. Kim et al. [57] compared postpartum depression rates in teen versus older mothers in a large Canadian sample (n = 6421). The prevalence of depression in the teen mothers in their sample, who were 15–19 years old, was 14% in the teen mothers compared to 7.2% in the adult mothers ($p < 0.001$). However, the overall rates of postpartum depression, at least in the USA, are probably much higher. Data from the Pregnancy Risk Assessment Monitoring System (PRAMS) of the Centers for Disease Control indicated a national rate of 13%, with rates by state ranging from 9.7 to 23.5%. The highest rate of postpartum depression (22.2%) was in women aged 19 years and younger. Elevated rates were also correlated with American Indian/Alaska Native race, smoking during or after pregnancy, intimate partner violence before or during pregnancy, self-reported depression before or during pregnancy, and death of an infant after birth [13]. These data point to the importance of age as well as social factors as risk factors for depression.

Even higher rates were found in a prospective cohort study that assessed depressive symptoms in adolescent women in Texas up to 4 years postpartum. This study, of nearly 1000 of a multicultural group of adolescents up to age 18 who gave birth at the University of Texas Medical Branch in Galveston Texas, found that 57% of teenage mothers had moderate to severe depression during the first postpartum year [86]. In comparison, CDC data indicated a rate of about 15% for adult women.

Data from other countries are consistent with these findings. A Portuguese study done several years ago compared 54 pregnant adolescents with 54 adult women during the third trimester of pregnancy and 2–3 months postpartum [35]. This study found that at both time points depressive symptoms as well as scores on the Edinburgh Postnatal Depression scale were considerably higher for the adolescent mothers (25.9% for adolescent mothers versus 11.1% for adult mothers during pregnancy, and 25.9% versus 9.3% postpartum). These differences held even when socio demographic factors were taken into account, suggesting that young age by itself is an important risk factor for depression during pregnancy and in the postpartum period.

Risk Factors

Prenatal depression is the strongest risk factor for postpartum depression in women of any age. Pregnancy itself, at least in adolescents, does not seem to increase the risk of depression. If childbearing adolescents are carefully compared with controls who are similar, the rates of depression are similar. This is illustrated by the findings of two reasonably large studies.

Hipwell and colleagues looked at the trajectories of depressive symptoms in 147 childbearing adolescents compared with a group of adolescents matched for SES and a variety of other variables who were not parents [45]. The two groups were similar with respect to age, living with a single parent, depression severity, having experienced sexual abuse, parenting or peer factors, social adversity, and neighborhood problems. Notably the two groups did not differ in terms of psychosocial adversity. There were no differences between the groups with respect to severity of depressive symptoms, and the teen mothers actually did better than the controls in some respects. Over time, during the pregnancy and afterwards, the teen mothers decreased their marijuana use compared to the controls, who tended to increase their use over the time of the study. Teen moms also had fewer conduct problems. The use of alcohol and tobacco did not change in either group. They concluded "the results do not support the notion that adolescent childbearing represents a period of heightened risk for depression or problem behaviors."

Another study compared pregnant (203) and nulliparous (188) adolescents in terms of levels of distress, mother–daughter relationship, and partner support. In this study adolescents were recruited from hospital clinics, community health care centers, and high school clinics serving predominantly economically disadvantaged communities in New Haven, Bridgeport, and Hartford, Connecticut. Both groups showed similarly elevated levels of distress compared to normative data for adolescents. However, some factors seemed to more negatively affect pregnant and parenting adolescents—a more distant mother–daughter relationship, lack of current partner support, and a history of physical maltreatment from adult family members [63].

These and other studies point to the importance of contextual factors in pre- and postpartum depression. Depression does not occur independently of social and cultural variables. Rates of pre- and postpartum depression are intertwined with the socio-economic conditions of the young women who become pregnant and give birth. Support from the adolescent's mother or the baby's father is an important protective factor, while overall stress level is a risk factor [12], as are family conflict, fewer social supports, and low self-esteem [81].

Milan and colleagues noted that physical maltreatment and lack of partner support were important determinants of depression for pregnant teens. Kim and colleagues in the study cited above [57] noted that teen mothers, in addition to having an increased prevalence of postpartum depression among teen mothers, also had less social support.

In summary, pregnancy by itself does not appear to increase the risk of depression. However, pregnancy in the context of adverse psychosocial conditions, conditions which are themselves associated with an increased risk of depression, does carry an increased risk. Given the association of teen pregnancy with adverse social conditions, the likelihood that pregnant teens will experience depressive episodes is significant.

Consequences

For Parents In addition to the morbidity and mortality of this disorder at the time of acute illness, it has multiple future consequences for those afflicted as well. For example, having depression may increase the likelihood of having a second pregnancy within 2 years of the first (Barnet & Liu). These subsequent pregnancies can lead to a perpetuation of poverty, lack of education, and further missed opportunities; only reinforcing the cycle in future generations.

For Children Untreated maternal depression increases the risk of preterm birth, small for gestational age babies, low birth weights, preeclampsia and spontaneous abortion [33]. Untreated maternal depression is also associated with increased negative-intrusive and hostile behavior, and decreased engaged and positive-sensitive behavior [61]. It is linked to poor attachment between mother and infant, delayed development of cognitive and linguistic skills, and increased risk for behavioral problems later in the child's life [71].

Subclinical depression is also a significant factor that negatively affects infant development, having similar effects as clinical depression on quality of attachment, hostility, and lack of pleasure in interaction [95]. Negative cognitions, decreased self-confidence, and a tendency to see infant affect as negative have all been found to be associated with this condition [14].

Treatment

The mainstays of treatment for depression are psychotherapy and antidepressant medication. Cognitive behavioral therapy (CBT) and interpersonal psychotherapy have been shown to be particularly effective in adolescents. CBT focuses on the identification and correction of cognitive distortions that are a crucial part of the depression. IPT focuses on identifying and improving problems in key relationships. Because of the importance of social support, interventions that focus on improving social support at home, school, and community are crucial. We will discuss these in the chapter on interventions.

Suicide and Suicidality

Suicide is the third leading cause of death during adolescence [65]. Adolescent suicide rates in the USA, which had leveled off and were essentially unchanged from 2000 to 2007, increased between 2007 and 2014, and increased dramatically, especially for girls, between 2014 and 2017. Suicide and suicidality are concerns during the vulnerable state of pregnancy [27]. Thus, we might expect it to be a particular concern for pregnant and parenting teens. Although, on the whole, suicide rates are lower for women who have given birth than for those who have not been pregnant, suicide is one of the leading causes of death in the year following delivery [76]. Suicide attempts may occur up to 9–12 months postpartum with mothers who had untreated psychiatric illness or suicidality in their pregnancy (ibid.), underscoring the need for close follow-up during this period.

Risk Factors

Major depressive disorder and other affected disorders are by far the main risk factors for suicide attempts and suicide; a history of suicidal ideation (the wish to die, thoughts of killing oneself, and the intent to kill oneself) are also important risk factors.

Younger maternal age is a significant risk factor for suicide. Studies have shown that pregnant adolescents have significantly higher rates of suicidality than pregnant adult women, i.e., 10–45% of adolescent mothers struggle with suicidal ideation at some point in their pregnancy [19, 38, 76]. Significant risk factors for suicidal behaviors among pregnant adolescents include major depressive disorder, physical and sexual abuse, prior abortions, lower socioeconomic class, poor education, and poor parental bonding styles [22].

Several psychiatric and social factors are known to be associated with suicidality in pregnant women. These include being younger, unmarried status, unemployment, previous abortion or intention to abort the current pregnancy, unintended pregnancy, low social support, intimate partner violence, and psychiatric disorders such as anxiety and depression. The prevalence of these risk factors among pregnant adolescents places them at high risk. The risk is compounded by the increased stress and social stigma associated with teen pregnancy.

In a study of 828 Brazilian adolescents who were receiving prenatal care in a public clinic, Coelho et al. [22] found suicidality to be related to adverse socioeconomic and psychosocial circumstances, including low education, low social support, and exposure to physical violence. Similar findings have been reported by others. As has been found with adults, previous abortion and intention to abort the current pregnancy were significantly associated with suicidality. Coelho et al. found the rate of suicidality was six times higher in pregnant adolescents with panic disorder after adjustment for all other variables, suggesting that pregnant teenagers with panic disorder are an especially vulnerable subgroup in terms of suicidal behavior [101].

Anxiety

Characteristics

Anxiety is a condition that involves excessive fear and worry, as well as physiological and behavioral manifestations. Fear is a reaction to a real or perceived imminent threat, whereas anxiety is the anticipation of future threat. Each has its own criteria and characteristics. Several types of anxiety are listed in the American Psychiatric Association's Diagnostic and Statistical Manual of Mental Disorders (DSM-5; [4]). These include generalized anxiety disorder (GAD), panic disorder (PD) with or without agoraphobia, social anxiety disorder, and specific phobia.

Although the disorders differ from each other in terms of the situations that cause fear and anxiety, and the cognitive ideation that goes along with the emotions, they all involve excessive fear and apprehensiveness. Anxiety is part of the human condition, but the anxiety of anxiety disorders is excessive and often crippling. It is often accompanied by physiological changes, such as elevated heart rate, and heightened cortisol secretion, which could affect fetal development. After delivery, anxiety can interfere with maternal infant bonding.

Prevalence

Anxiety disorders are the most common psychiatric disorders among adolescents. In what is generally considered the most valid and reliable study on prevalence of psychiatric disorders in adolescence Kessler and colleagues (2012) found the 12-month prevalence of any anxiety disorder among adolescents was 24.9% [56]. Given this prevalence, and the fact that preexisting anxiety disorders are the strongest risk factors for perinatal anxiety disorders, we might expect these disorders to be highly prevalent among teen parents. However, data on this are sparse, as studies of anxiety disorders in pregnant and parenting adolescents are almost non-existent. Nonetheless, many studies of pregnant women and new parents include older adolescents, so the findings are probably relevant. In this section, we review the literature on anxiety disorders in pregnancy in general and consider how what we know about this disorder may apply to young parents.

During Pregnancy In their review of studies published between 1990 and 2013, Siegel and Brandon [89] found only 1 study that examined the prevalence of self-reported anxiety and stress in pregnant adolescents [5]. This study used the State-Trait Anxiety Inventory, a widely used questionnaire that has norms for various ages and populations. Scores from a sample of 120 pregnant teenagers were compared with norms for this instrument. The scores for both state and trait anxiety were higher among the pregnant teens; levels of state anxiety, a more transient condition, differed more than trait anxiety between the two groups. The authors did not use diagnostic tools but measured affective symptoms using self-report questionnaires. They reported that 35% of their sample felt "very upset, tense, or upset" "often" or "very often." While this study cannot provide information about the prevalence of actual disorders, it does suggest that levels of anxiety are elevated in pregnant teens. Unfortunately, this seems to be the only study that focused exclusively on adolescents. Other studies of anxiety among pregnant women are mainly concerned with adults, although many do include older adolescents.

In a review of adult studies published 5 years after the review by Siegel and Brandon cited above, Viswasman and colleagues [103] conducted a comprehensive literature search and meta-analysis, finding 36 studies of the prevalence, onset and course of anxiety disorders during pregnancy. They found that the rates reported in these studies were extremely variable. For example, prevalence rates for generalized anxiety disorder (GAD) varied between 9% and 22.9%; those for specific phobia (SP) from 3.2 to 19.9%; for social anxiety disorder (SAD) 2–27%, and for post-traumatic stress disorder (PTSD), 6–16%. When compared to what is known about prevalence rates for women in the general population, they concluded rates for GAD SP, PTSD were lower among pregnant women, but OCD and panic disorder were more common [103]. There are many reasons for the variable results obtained in these studies. Most studies do not separate anxiety into different subtypes. The criteria used for diagnosis vary in terms of instruments and cutoff points. Time frames of studies are variable, and samples are often convenience samples or otherwise not representative.

In the Postpartum Period Postpartum anxiety is common among women in general, although its prevalence among adolescent mothers is unknown. In a narrative review of studies published from 2010 to 2017, Field found prevalence rates of 13–40%, much higher than the previously reported rates of between 2.2% and 8.8% [34]. For example, Tietz and colleagues, interviewing mothers when their infants were 4 months old found 30 of 78 mothers in their German sample had postpartum anxiety disorders without depression when interviewed [96]. A Canadian study that used diagnostic interviews for women who scored above cutoff points on self-report questionnaires found the prevalence of anxiety symptomatology at 1, 4, and 8 weeks postpartum to be 22.6%, 17.2%, and 14.8%, respectively [26]. Fairbrother et al. [31] found both prenatal and postpartum anxiety to be more prevalent than depression in a study of 310 women in Vancouver. This study used diagnostic interviews for participants who scored above cutoff scores on questionnaires. The prevalence of any anxiety disorder during pregnancy and the early postpartum period was 15.8% and 17.1%, respectively, and exceeded that of depression (3.9% and 4.8%, respectively). Slightly less than 5% of participants were comorbid for both an anxiety disorder and depression.

Risk Factors

The evidence from studies of populations that include older adolescents indicates that prenatal anxiety is associated with younger maternal age as well as unplanned pregnancy, suggesting that young parents are at higher risk.

Anxiety tends to be a chronic condition, waxing and waning according to changes in life circumstances, stressful events, and so on. Given the life-altering nature of pregnancy, childbirth, and motherhood it is not surprising that these experiences would be associated with some anxiety as a normative experience. For most women this anxiety is not disabling and can be growth-promoting and lead to adaptive responses, such as seeking social support.

As with other disorders, prior history is an important risk factor. Women who are prone to worry anyway are likely to have increased levels of anxiety during their pregnancies. Martini and colleagues [62] followed women recruited from outpatient settings from early in their pregnancies until 16 months after delivery. They found pre-existing diagnoses to have the strongest correlations with both prepartum and postpartum anxiety, with p levels less than 0.001 [62]. Having experienced trauma prior to pregnancy was correlated with anxiety disorders during the pregnancy but not afterwards. The authors found a variety of trajectories–some disorders actually remitted during pregnancy, while others have new onset, and still others recurred or were exacerbated. They also found psychosocial factors were important, including self-esteem and social support. In the case of some disorders, it is possible to tie the onset of the disorder with specific concerns about pregnancy and parenting. For example, panic disorder tended to be most prevalent during the third trimester as delivery approached. This is especially true for women contemplating Caesarian section.

A French study of 400 women attending a prenatal clinic looked at anxiety and coping strategies in the third trimester and 2 months postpartum. On the basis of self-report questionnaires this study found high rates of anxiety both antenatally (18.8%) and postpartum (20.2%). Comparing anxious with non-anxious women, the authors found the anxious women tended to blame themselves and deny reality, well those without anxiety used adaptive coping mechanisms such as reframing, acceptance, and humor [41]. Although this study only included women aged 19 and older, there was a tendency toward more anxiety among the younger women. The authors noted that rates of anxiety were twice as high as those reported in other studies for depression, and concluded that perinatal anxiety is a major health issue.

Consequences

For Mothers The mechanisms through which anxiety operates on mother–child interactions are not very well understood. They might involve perceptions of cues from infants, avoidance of the infants, or inappropriate responses to infants. One study showed that mothers with generalized anxiety disorder had difficulty correctly identifying happy faces of infants from pictures [9]. Another study showed anxious mothers, when videotaped interacting with their infants, showed less sensitive responding and reduced emotional tone than did mothers without anxiety [73]. This was true even when mothers with comorbid depression were excluded from the data analysis.

Maternal anxiety has also been associated with intrusive interactions and parenting behavior [23]. Feldman and colleagues [32] did a prospective study on mother–infant dyads at 6 months, comparing adult women who had postpartum depression or anxiety with each other and with a third group with no symptoms using various structured assessment instruments as well as home visits and videotaped sessions. They were interested in looking at infants' social engagement, fear regulation, and physiological stress reactivity as measured by cortisol levels. Consistent with other literature maternal depression had the largest negative effect on infants. But anxiety also was associated with problems. While the anxious mothers did interact with their infants socially as much as those without any disorder, their interactions tended to be intrusive and not well adapted to the infants' cues.

One significant deleterious impact of postnatal anxiety is on breastfeeding, as Tietz and colleagues found in the study cited above (2014). They found mothers with post-natal anxiety were less likely to initiate breast feeding, and more likely to have difficulties with breast feeding and terminate breast feeding. A systematic review confirmed these findings and also found women with postpartum anxiety were more likely to supplement with formula in the hospital; there was even some evidence of negative effects on breast milk composition [26].

For Children Anxiety has biological correlates that can affect overall health and functioning and could affect fetal development. Both fear and anxiety are associated with activation of the autonomic nervous system and the neuroendocrine systems. Fear is accompanied by physiological changes related to surges of autonomic arousal, such as elevated heart rate. Anxiety is accompanied by muscle tension and vigilance in preparation for future danger and cautious or avoidant behaviors. Alterations in neuroendocrine functioning associated with anxiety have the potential to affect fetal development. After delivery, anxiety can interfere with maternal infant bonding, possibly because of the avoidant behavior that frequently accompanies it.

Unlike the case with other disorders, prenatal anxiety is not clearly related to obstetric complications. There do seem to be significant postnatal effects on children in many cases, including problems with bonding [21]. However, the evidence for postnatal effects is not as clear cut as it is for depression. Since anxiety is so often comorbid with depression it is difficult to disentangle the effects of one from the other. This probably accounts for the inconsistent results of studies examining links between anxiety and mother–infant relationships. For example, Tietz and colleagues [52], in a study of a German sample of mother–infant dyads, found adverse effects of post-natal maternal anxiety on mother–infant interactions and infant temperament. However, when the data were analyzed with depressive symptoms controlled for, the relationship between anxiety disorders and mother-–infant bonding was nonsignificant. Although mothers with major depressive disorder were excluded from this study, many had subclinical depressive symptoms. The authors speculated that the anxious mothers' subclinical depression and/or avoidance of anxiety-provoking situations might have been the main reason for poor mother–infant bonding, rather than the anxiety disorders per se.

Treatment

The approach to management of anxiety during pregnancy is similar to that of depression and SSRIs are currently considered a first-line pharmacologic treatment for anxiety spectrum illness. Selective serotonin reuptake inhibitors are effective for anxiety and can be used safely during pregnancy [58]. Psychotherapy, especially cognitive behavioral therapy, has a strong evidence base in adolescents as well as adults. Reviewing treatments specifically for pregnant women and new parents, Nillni et al. [74] found CBT, as well as mindfulness-based therapy and exposure therapy, both forms of CBT, to be efficacious. Benzodiazepines are effective in reducing anxiety symptoms, but their use is limited by risk of abuse and adverse effect profiles. Physical activity can reduce symptoms of GAD and PD. Evidence is emerging for the efficacy of complementary and alternative treatments.

Summary

In summary, postpartum anxiety can negatively affect the quality of the mother–infant interaction. Anxiety-prone individuals tend to view changes and new demands with apprehension. One of the key symptoms of anxiety disorders is avoidance. Mothers' avoidance of anxiety-provoking situations may account for the effects of anxiety on mother–infant interactions. Other mediating factors might be lower self-esteem and self-confidence, and difficulty attuning to infants' emotional cues.

In light of the serious impairment in parental functioning and negative effects on infant development associated with anxiety disorders, it seems reasonable to recommend routine screening and active intervention for anxiety both in the prenatal and postnatal period. Although many guidelines have called for depression screening to be done routinely in obstetrical care, until recently there were no such formal recommendations for anxiety. In 2018, the American Psychiatric Association included anxiety disorders in a position statement that recommended screening by "physicians across all specialties to better detect, diagnose, and treat mood and anxiety disorders in pregnant and postpartum women." The fact that many of the instruments used to detect depression also include assessment of anxiety means that the amount of time spent on screening does not necessarily have to increase. We will discuss these later in this chapter.

Obsessive Compulsive Disorder

Characteristics

Obsessive compulsive disorder (OCD) is a disorder characterized by the presence of disabling obsessions and/or compulsions [4]. Obsessions, according to the DSM, are "recurrent and persistent thoughts, urges, or impulses that are experienced, at some time during the disturbance, as intrusive and unwanted, and that in most individuals cause marked anxiety or distress." The DSM adds, "The individual attempts to ignore or suppress such thoughts, urges, or images, or to neutralize them with some thought or action (i.e., by performing a compulsion)."

Compulsions are defined as "repetitive behaviors (e.g., hand washing, ordering, checking) or mental acts (e.g., praying, counting, repeating words silently) that the individual feels driven to perform in response to an obsession or according to rules that must be applied rigidly."

Symptoms of OCD often center around concerns about harming others. Obsessive-compulsive disorders in the postpartum period are commonly related to fears about harm befalling the child. Typical worries in perinatal OCD involve the infant's death during sleep, or of committing harm by shaking or stabbing the child, leaving the child alone in the bathtub, or misplacing the child. These may lead to excessive checking on a sleeping infant, or even to avoiding the baby for fear of inadvertently harming her. These thoughts are intrusive, distressing, and accompanied by anxiety. The child is not actually in danger, as there is great fear of the thoughts and of acting upon them [30]. The thoughts are recognized as irrational (in contrast to psychotic disorders).

Obsessions and compulsions without actual OCD are common during pregnancy and in the postpartum period. Miller and colleagues [64] found 37.5% of the women they screened to have subclinical obsessions or compulsions (compared to 11.2% who screened positive for OCD). The normal concerns of an expectant or new mother about the welfare of her child may shade into obsessions about the child's wellbeing or unwanted intrusive thoughts of hurting the newborn [72]. Indeed, such worries are present in significant numbers of women with no psychiatric condition [50]. Abramowitz and colleagues, using surveys mailed to childbearing women and partners, found 65% of respondents acknowledged intrusive thoughts [2]. This study was limited by a low response rate (only one fifth of a sample of 300 responded). Fairbrother and Woody found postpartum intrusive thoughts of accidental harm to the infant were universal, and unwanted thoughts of intentionally harming their infant were present in close to half of the sample (n = 100) they studied using questionnaires and structured interviews. Intrusive thoughts were increased in the presence of stress and low social support—conditions prevalent among young parents [30].

Although OCD typically has a gradual onset, when it occurs during the perinatal period, onset is often quite sudden, with rapid progression in severity [18]. When it occurs in the postpartum period its onset is usually occurs within the first 4 weeks of delivery. Comorbidity with depression and anxiety is common [8, 64]. Depression often involves obsessive rumination, and it has been suggested that OCD symptoms might be a component of a depressive illness. Comorbidity with eating disorders has also been reported [68].

Risk Factors

Pre-existing OCD one of the risk factors, but there are others. Zambaldi and colleagues followed a nonclinical sample of 400 women from the time they were 2 weeks postpartum until 26 weeks. They found OCD to be more prevalent among those who had a previous psychiatric history, somatic disease, had obstetrical complications, or were multiparous [105]. The type of pre-existing psychiatric disorder was not identified. Comorbidity with depression was common.

House and colleagues, in a prospective study that followed 56 women from their pregnancies through 1 year after delivery, found an association of OCD with younger age and Caesarian section deliveries, but not with specific obstetric or neonatal complications [47].

Neurobiological and Psychological Factors

Pregnancy and the postpartum period involve major hormonal changes, and these have been considered as possible etiological factors in perinatal OCD. A recent comprehensive review concluded that the evidence suggests it is likely that the dramatic changes in oxytocin, estrogen, and progesterone that occur in the puerperium are involved in OCD in the postpartum period [91]. These hormones regulate expression of various neural receptors and are also involved in the synthesis and release of neurotransmittors; changing hormone levels can have disregulatory effects on the serotonergic, dopaminergic, and glutaminergic neurotransmitter systems.

An alternative, and probably complementary, hypothesis is that cognitive factors play an important role in the genesis and maintenance of postpartum OCD. Interestingly OCD occurs in new fathers as well [1, 66] and has very similar symptoms to OCD in new mothers. Abramowitz and colleagues emphasize the importance of cognitive factors in OCD, pointing out that, given that new fathers are not subject to the same hormonal changes as mothers are, these changes cannot be involved in their symptoms, and there must be a psychological explanation. In new parents, particularly those who are first time parents, an exaggerated sense of responsibility, together with a tendency to overestimate threats, and misinterpretation of intrusive thoughts coalesce to give rise to obsessions about harm befalling children. In a prospective study, Abramowitz et al. [3] were able to demonstrate that prenatal scores on a questionnaire, the Obsessive Beliefs Inventory, predicted postpartum OCD.

Prevalence

OCD is a fairly common disorder in the general population—with a prevalence of 2–3% [55]. The peak age of onset is in the mid-20s for women (it is younger for men) [83].

There is evidence of higher rates of OCD with pregnancy and the postpartum period when asked retrospectively about the onset of OCD, substantial numbers of women identify childbirth as a precipitating event [83, 85, 100]. OCD onset is common during the peripartum period; Miller and colleagues found 52 of 461 women they screened (11.2%) screened positive for OCD [64]. Risk factors include prior OCD, Cesarean section, and miscarriage [17].

Consequences

For Mothers Unlike OCD outside of the perinatal period, perinatal OCD tends to be self-limited and usually does not progress to compulsions and chronicity, although in some cases it can become chronic. It causes considerable distress to affected individuals and their families. OCD does not appear to adversely affect pregnancy; House and colleagues found that there was actually a higher frequency of fetal loss among women without OCD than among those with the disorder, and no other adverse effects on the developing fetus have been found [47].

For Children The manifestations of this disorder can seriously adversely affect the parent–child relationship. Of particular concern is its impact on the parent–infant relationship and the family as a whole. Challacome and Wroe reported seeing cases in general practice in which children were removed from their homes because of parents' reports of intrusive thoughts of harming their infants, which healthcare personnel failed to realize were symptoms of OCD [18].

Treatment

The mainstays of treatment are serotonin reuptake inhibitors [99] and cognitive behavioral therapy (CBT). We discuss medication management of psychiatric disorders in a separate section. CBT for parents with OCD [29] involves three basic components: (1) psychoeducation about the ubiquity of the intrusive thoughts concerning harm to the infant; (2) exposure and response prevention (ERP); and cognitive restructuring. Patients are reassured that their thoughts are common and normal. Then, under the guidance of a therapist they are helped to expose themselves to their anxiety-provoking thoughts or situations (for example, a parent who avoids scissors for fear of cutting her infant is taught to hold scissors when sitting by herself. Response prevention refers to choosing not to engage in compulsive behavior (limiting the amount of time checking on a sleeping infant, for example). Patients are taught to carry out these activities on their own. Cognitive restructuring counters the false appraisals of risk or the belief that thoughts are equivalent to actions.

Post-Traumatic Stress Disorder (PTSD)

Characteristics

Posttraumatic stress disorder (PTSD) is a complex psychiatric disorder involving (1) exposure to a traumatic event(s) and (2) a constellation of symptoms involving intrusive symptoms—such as memories, dreams, and dissociative reactions or flashbacks. There is intense distress at reminders of the traumatic event(s), leading to avoidance of triggering situations which resemble some aspect of the original trauma. PTSD is accompanied by alterations in cognitive functioning—such as lack of memory for aspects of the trauma and negative distortions in the appraisal of oneself and others [4].

PTSD is a pre-existing condition for some teens who become pregnant, while for others the pregnancy itself and childbirth may be experienced as traumatic, particularly if the pregnancy and delivery are complicated. Postpartum PTSD is particularly likely if there are fears about childbirth, complications to the pregnancy and delivery, or if the childbirth experience is unusually painful. As we have discussed in the chapter on trauma and adolescent pregnancy, physical and sexual abuse, intimate partner violence, and community interpersonal violence are prevalent in the lives of young women who have unplanned pregnancies. In some cases, the pregnancy itself is a result of sexual assault, while in other cases, teens who have experienced sexual abuse or other emotional trauma in their lives become pregnant. There is a high degree of comorbidity with PTSD, especially with depression, anxiety and substance use disorders [88].

Prevalence

There have been few studies of the prevalence of PTSD among pregnant and parenting adolescents. The prevalence of PTSD in the general population is about 3–5%. Prevalence rates vary considerably among various subsets, with rates highest among low-income populations—the same group that has the highest rates of teen pregnancy. The few studies that have compared younger and older pregnant women within the same demographic category have found prevalence rates to be higher in younger pregnant and parenting women—around 10%, with women 19 years old or younger having a 2 1/2 times greater likelihood of having current PTSD compared with those older than 19 [67, 94]. Tabet and colleagues actually found PTSD to be more common than major depressive disorder among the young women they studied. The prevalence of postpartum PTSD is higher—as high as 16%—in at risk samples, which include women with histories of psychiatric illness or trauma [43].

Risk Factors

We know that people who have experienced past trauma are more likely to be retraumatized by subsequent adverse events, so a previous history of trauma is one of the main risk factors.

Younger age of childbearing is also risk factor [87], probably because women who have experienced trauma are at higher risk for early pregnancy. Other risk factors include a history of any psychiatric illness and high risk pregnancy. A meta-analysis of studies on postpartum PTSD among adult women found a prevalence of almost 16% among high risk samples, as opposed to 3% in community samples [43]. An interesting small study found avoidant attachment styles to be a risk [11]. Although this study involved older women, and may not be applicable to young mothers, difficulties with trust are part of the avoidant style, and might be expected to be prevalent among teen mothers in care environments that do not foster acceptance and support.

In general, having a mental illness increases the risk of experiencing trauma, and trauma increases the risk of developing psychological symptoms and mental disorders.

PTSD is postulated to result from various alterations in neuroendocrine and neural functioning, which in turn affect the contextualization of experience and emotional responses. These alterations are fueled by exposure to traumatic events and the ensuing emotional and physiological responses.

Consequences

For Mothers PTSD has a significant impact on most areas of daily functioning, including interpersonal relationships, ability to function at work or at school, and quality of life [49]. Brain imaging studies show alterations in the hippocampus, and impaired connectivity in the frontoparietal regions. These are believed to be responsible for the impairment in executive functioning and emotional regulation that is at the core of PTSD [88].

For Children In addition to causing significant disability for affected individuals, PTSD can have major adverse effects on the mother–child relationship. While teasing out the effects of PTSD from those of depression or anxiety is problematic as these conditions so often occur together, it does seem that PTSD significantly increases the likelihood of negative parenting, characterized by higher levels of avoidance, intrusiveness, hostility, controlling and overprotective behavior, and less sensitivity, responsivity, and emotional availability [20]. Attachment-based trauma in particular seems to interfere with prenatal attachment. Maternal disengagement and dissociation can be triggered by the infant's distress, leading to reduced responsivity and sensitivity.

Treatment Screening pregnant adolescents and new mothers for PTSD in primary care settings has been recommended by the American Academy of Pediatrics [46]. There are two short questionnaires—a 4-item screen designed specifically for primary care settings (the PC-PTSD; [78]) and a 17-item checklist, the PCL, which exists in various versions [16]. A version of the PCL has been validated in pregnant women [40]. In addition to being a screening instrument it also quantifies the severity of symptoms and can be used to monitor the response to treatment.

The goal of treatment is reduction in the severity of disabling symptoms and improved emotional regulation. Psychosocial interventions, including mindfulness, cognitive restructuring, and trauma-specific desensitization approaches, such as exposure therapy, involve psychoeducation and a focus on emotion regulation and cognitive processing [88].

The recognition of the important impact the trauma has on survivors' receptivity and responsivity to services in a variety of public sector settings—health, social services, and educational settings—has led to the concepts of trauma-informed care and trauma sensitive services. The focus is on understanding a person's behavior in terms of his or her past traumatic experiences, and taking care not to re-traumatize the individual in interactions and policies and procedures. In the USA, a National Center for trauma-informed care (NCTIC) provides guidance about implementing Trauma-informed services [93].

Trauma-informed cognitive behavioral therapy has a strong evidence base. This treatment may involve exposure and desensitization, in which a person is taught relaxation techniques such as deep breathing and then in the context of psychotherapeutic support is helped to recall aspects of a traumatic event. Over time and with repetition, the patient is able to recall these things with attenuated emotional reactions and decreased avoidance. Eye movement desensitization and reprocessing (EMDR) is an innovative treatment in which the patient recalls traumatic images while engaging in horizontal eye movement. Other innovative treatments include transcranial magnetic stimulation and biofeedback. These are all described in a publicationication by the Substance Abuse and Mental Health Services Administration (SAMHSA) [93]. Antidepressant medications can also be helpful in reducing symptoms, but do not seem to produce long lasting remission. Only two have been approved by the FDA for treatment of PTSD, paroxetine and sertraline. A wide variety of others are used to deal with symptoms of anxiety and insomnia.

Bipolar Disorder

Bipolar disorder (BD) has its onset prior to adulthood in over half of cases, with over a third starting during adolescence [59]. Moreover, pregnancy is associated with a high risk of recurrence in women who have a history of bipolar disorder [90]. A woman who has a history of bipolar disorder is highly likely to have a mood episode during pregnancy, and even more likely to have one during the postpartum period. Mood episodes are significantly more common during the first month postpartum than during pregnancy [6]. In mothers with bipolar disorder the incidence of mood episodes within 3 months of giving birth ranges from 25 to 79% [84].

BD also carries with it a risk of unplanned pregnancy. In addition to mood disturbances, BD symptoms include impulsive behavior, poor judgment, and hypersexuality, each of which might lead affected adolescents to engage in high risk sexual behavior, putting them at risk for pregnancy. Vigod and colleagues in their large population-based study of teenagers in Toronto found that a substantial proportion of unplanned pregnancy occurred in adolescents with bipolar disorder [102]. Their research confirmed the findings of earlier clinical studies that showed high rates of teenage pregnancy among girls with bipolar disorder. For example, Hefner and colleagues, in their prospective follow-up study of 23 adolescents who had had a manic episode found that 30% had at least one unplanned pregnancy by the age of 20 [44]. In comparison, the rate for a comparison group of girls in the 15–19 age range in the same local area was less than 1%. Another study of a larger group (249) of adolescents found a 5% 12-month prevalence of pregnancy and abortion in this group [42]. The prevalence was even greater in those adolescents who had substance abuse disorders in addition to their bipolar disorder—20% became pregnant and 12% had abortions.

The Course and Outcome of Bipolar Youth (COBY) study was a multisite multiyear longitudinal study that involved over 400 youth, and looked at a number of risk factors and outcome variables over a mean time of 10 years [15]). One component of the study involved exploring sexual risk behaviors, including young age at first sexual activity, unprotected sex, and multiple partners. Hypomania (as opposed to depression or mixed mania and depression) was identified as carrying the highest risk for sexual risk behavior.

Consequences

For Mothers Bipolar disorder is associated with a number of risks to the person affected. These most notably include suicide [84], substance misuse [42] and psychosis. Pregnant women with BD are also at risk for gestational hypertension and antepartum hemorrhage.

For Children Children born to mothers with bipolar disorder are at risk for prematurity, low birth weight, and small size for gestational age [84]. They may also have impaired stress responsivity and physiological regulation [51]. A slightly increased risk of congenital abnormalities (around 4% compared with 3% in the total population) has also been reported; this may be due to treatment with certain mood stabilizers, such as valproic acid, which are known to be associated with congenital abnormalities [84].

Radke-Yarrow and colleagues found children of mothers with bipolar disorder were more likely to be insecurely attached to their mothers than were children of mothers with unipolar depression [79]. Since depression has significant adverse effects on mother–infant bonding, it appears bipolar disorder poses an even more significant risk. Responsiveness to infants involves sensitivity to and accurate perception of infant cues, appropriate responses, and reciprocity, as we have discussed in the chapter on infant development. Ideally interactions are dyadically synchronous—the mother responds to the baby's communications and the baby responds to the mother's emotional tone as expressed by her voice, facial expressions and other actions. They form a dyad and are tuned in to each other. This synchrony fosters emotional regulation in the infant. In the case of depression, mothers tend to be unable to respond. With bipolar disorder, although mothers are responsive and interactive, they have difficulty interpreting their infants' cues, thus impairing dyadic coordination and synchronicity [6]. In addition, they seem to have more negative affect than healthy controls (ibid).

Assessment and Treatment

While some patients will present with a previous diagnosis of bipolar disorder, especially if there have been frank manic episodes, it is often missed in general medical settings [24]. This is especially the case with adolescents, who tend to present with depression initially. In particular, the presence of psychotic symptoms with depression in adolescence may be a harbinger of bipolar disorder. Screening for depression should also include an assessment of past manic symptoms. The Mood Disorder Questionnaire is a simple and widely validated instrument that includes questions about manic symptoms and has been used for adolescents as well as adults in primary care settings [104].

Mood stabilizing medication is the mainstay of treatment of bipolar disorder. Because of concerns about teratogenicity, there is often a reluctance to prescribe mood stabilizers, but the risks associated with untreated bipolar disorder during pregnancy are sufficiently high to warrant treatment. Lithium has a history of efficacy in the perinatal period and the general consensus is that patients who have had a good response to it should be continued on it with careful monitoring. Twice daily dosing is recommended to reduce the peak levels of concentration and thereby reduce fetal exposure [27]. Discontinuation from the onset of labor until after delivery is also recommended .The main concern with lithium is a fetal heart valve anomality known as Ebstein's anomaly, but this condition appears to be quite rare – 1 in 1000 compared to 1 in 20,000 in the general population [75].

Lamotragine, an antiepileptic medication, is an alternative. It has been well studied in pregnant patients with epilepsy and appears to have no significant teratogenic effects [75]. Other anticonvulsants, such as valproic acid and carbamazepine are known to have significant teratogenic effects. Electroconvulsive therapy, although rarely used, is safe and effective [27].

Psychotic Disorders

Characteristics

Psychoses are not psychiatric diagnoses per se but rather the term is used to refer to a group of severe mental disorders that involve psychotic symptoms as well as significant impairments in day-to-day functioning. Disorders associated with psychotic symptoms include schizophrenia, bipolar disorder, brief psychotic disorder, schizophreniform disorder, and psychoses associated with substance abuse or metabolic or endocrine disorders [4]. They are sometimes divided into affective and non-affective psychoses.

Psychotic symptoms can involve distorted perceptions (hallucinations and delusions), disorganized and aberrant thinking (ideas of reference, grandiosity, delusions), disorganized behavior and illogical speech patterns. Delusions involve fixed false beliefs. Grandiose delusions, for example, may include a belief that one is God or sent by God, persecutory delusions that there is a plot against oneself, or hypochondriacal delusions, such as convictions about the body rotting or illness.

The various psychotic disorders can be differentiated from each other based on duration, dysfunction, associated substance use, bizarreness of delusions, and presence of depression or mania. These disorders are relatively rare, with prevalence of between 1.5 and 3.5% in the general population.The peak age of onset is in during late adolescence and early adulthood. While some cases of psychosis among pregnant and parenting women predate their pregnancy, others appear de novo in the postpartum period, and are termed postpartum psychoses, a term that includes any psychotic illness occurring in the first 12 months after delivery.

Schizophrenia is typically an illness of young adulthood. The full blown illness is often preceded by a prodromal period of subsyndromal symptoms, sometimes referred to as attenuated psychoses. This prodromal period can be several years in duration, often beginning during adolescence. While the signs and symptoms associated with full blown psychosis are fairly easily recognized, prodromal states are often unrecognized and may even masquerade as other disorders, such as conduct disorder [36]. In many cases there is a long prodromal period between the onset of first symptoms and the recognition of the disorder. Both prospective and retrospective studies have shown that the length of time from when early symptoms such as delusional thinking and mild hallucinations appear to when the disorder becomes manifest averages several years [101]. Early symptoms frequently go unrecognized, causing delays in treatment that may have grave consequences for prognosis.

Drug use can produce psychotic symptoms in vulnerable individuals. Often these are transient and will dissipate with cessation of use. Amphetamines and cannabis are most often involved. Cannabis-induced psychotic states severe enough to warrant inpatient treatment are often early signs of schizophrenia disorder [101].

Prevalence

Vigod and colleagues' found evidence that having a psychotic disorder as an adolescent increases the risk for pregnancy [102]. They found 30% of the girls with major mental illness who gave birth in the group they studied had a primary psychotic disorder (795 of the total group of 71,098 or about 1%). This is in contrast with the data for adult women with psychotic disorders, who are less likely to get pregnant and to bear children than those without these illnesses, even those with non-psychotic mental illnesses [48]. Vigod and colleagues have noted [102] "Preventive programs in most developed countries have not focused explicitly on mental health as a risk factor, which may partly explain why fertility rates are not decreasing as rapidly in this group."

Howard and colleagues looked at records from a primary care database that included women as young as 15. They found in general women with psychotic disorders had markedly lower fertility rates (measured by recorded births) than a matched cohort of without these disorders, but this was not true for women under 25. Although they had a small number of pregnant women with psychotic disorders in the 15–19-year-old age group, this group actually had higher fertility rates than did the comparison group; with a fertility rate that was 1.41 times the rate of non-affected women of the same age. The rate for women aged 20–24 was less than that of the comparison group, but the difference was less fin this age group than it was for the older groups [48].

Schizophrenia is not a single entity but rather a group of conditions that are phenotypically similar. Current evidence supports a multifactorial etiology, with both biological and environmental factors being involved. Biological factors include genetic risk factors, perinatal insults and birth complications, and cannabis use. Childhood trauma is also implicated [77].

Schizophrenia is currently viewed as a primarily neurodevelopmental disorder, an outcome of gene–environment interactions, with alterations in brain development being demonstrable on neuroimaging studies [28]. Brain imaging studies have implicated insufficient synaptic pruning and faulty myelination, and alterations in neurotransmitters [77]. That genetics is an important factor, but not the only factor, is indicated by the 40–50% concordance rate in identical twins [39].

Consequences

For Mothers Psychotic disorders can have major adverse effects on parenting. In part this is due to impairment in day-to-day functioning, with depression and all its concomitants playing a role, and in part due to psychotic symptoms themselves, which interfere with thinking, attention and focus. In extreme (fortunately rare) cases, parents may have delusions and command hallucinations telling them to harm their infants. Mothers with psychotic disorders often notice these impairments. A qualitative study that explored parents' own perceptions of how their psychotic disorder affected their parenting found the parents were aware of and concerned about their illness interfering with their ability to effectively parent [92].

For Children In the past it was usual for children of mothers with psychotic disorders to be placed outside the home. This was in part due to a general assumption that such women cannot provide adequate care for their children. The approach now is to assess competency to care and decide what resources need to be in place to help the woman parent.

Having a disorder that causes severe impairments in cognitive functioning would seem to put interfere in a major way with parent–child relationships. There have been numerous attempts to study how mothers with psychotic illnesses interact with their infants. Many of these observational studies have occurred on mother baby units, which exist primarily in Western European countries as well as in Australia These units provide opportunities for careful observation of mother–child interactions and for the implementation of interventions designed to improve the interactions. Studies have been done comparing women with psychotic disorders with those with affective disorders, usually depression. Ramsauer and colleagues [80] conducted a systematic review of studies of the impact of postpartum psychosis on infants. Although the methodologies and selection criteria varied considerably among the studies, there was a fair amount of convergence in the problems they identified. These included mothers' difficulties identifying and discriminating affective states, odd or unusual responses to infants, and problems with the affective tone of communications. A particular concern is maternal hostility, which is an indicator of seriously impaired mother–child interaction.

Another systematic review that looked specifically at schizophrenia concluded that mothers diagnosed with schizophrenia showed reduced social contact, greater tension, and more behavioral intrusiveness versus controls during the first 12 months, as compared to affective and nonclinical controls [25].

Treatment

Prompt treatment of psychotic disorders is crucial. There is good evidence that delaying treatment has an adverse effect on prognosis, and appropriate treatment of the first episode is particularly important. Antipsychotic medications in combination with psychosocial treatment are the mainstays of treatment. Measures to enhance adherence to treatment through psychoeducation, psychological and social support, family involvement, and case management are crucial [101]. With appropriate medical treatment and community-based care, remission rates of about 80% can be achieved in schizophrenia, especially with early treatment during first episodes [107].

Although in the past the presence of a psychotic disorder would have been considered grounds for termination of pregnancy or relinquishing of custody for the baby, as treatment options have improved and as the recognition that the prognosis in psychotic disorders is not uniformly grim, attitudes have shifted towards supporting mothers and children rather than separating them.

Mother–baby units offer an opportunity for mothers to receive treatment for their illness while their interactions with their infants can be closely monitored. Importantly, many studies have noted improvement in maternal behavior and mother–infant bonding during the stay in the mother baby units [80].

A major concern for parents with a history of psychotic illness is the possibility that they will need to be hospitalized because of a recurrence. or that they will lose custody of their children. While in some cases this may be necessary, having a psychotic disorder is not necessarily a contraindication to being a good parent. These disorders, once considered a reason for long-term institutionalization, no longer have such a dismal prognosis. Newer medications, especially second generation antipsychotic medications, can produce long-term remissions, especially in younger patients whose treatment is begun early. Psychosocial support is essential, as is adherence to treatment. Long acting forms of antipsychotic medications are available that improve adherence and outcomes. Families are key, as they often have varying degrees of responsibility for child care.

Several parameters need to be assessed in order to determine parental competency. These include a willingness to adhere to treatment, the ability to self-monitor, and the availability of surrogate caretakers. Wraparound services—intensive, individualized care involving a variety of interventions—can be helpful [53]. Typically, wraparound includes a person who works with various service providers to develop a plan of care, coordinates the services provided and monitors outcomes, making adjustments as needed over time. It is designed to avoid the fragmentation that can arise when multiple agencies are involved. In the case of infants and young children, the wraparound team would most likely involve family members, child protective services, pediatricians, and mental health professionals including psychiatrists The focus of wraparound is on identifying strengths and responding to families' perceptions of their needs and preferences. Cultural competence is one of its core values.

Summary

In summary, pregnant and parenting teens have higher rates of psychiatric disorders than older women. However, the higher prevalence can be accounted for by factors other than the pregnancy per se. First, adolescents who become parents are more likely that those who do not to have pre-existing mental health problems such as depression, trauma histories, bipolar disorder, and substance misuse; these conditions place them at risk for becoming pregnant. In addition, teen parents are likely to be members of marginalized minorities, live in disadvantaged environments, and experience a variety of adverse life events. All of these things are risk factors for psychiatric disorders. Thus, the same factors that underlie elevated rates of mental disorder also predispose to early unplanned pregnancy. These facts have important implications for interventions and social policy, which we will discuss in subsequent chapters.

The presence of a psychiatric illness adds another layer of complexity to the medical and psychosocial care of the pregnant and parenting teenager. However, good treatments are available, and the field of perinatal psychiatry has grown and developed, with several published reviews and guidelines to aid practitioners, including one specifically focused on adolescents [37]. The Centers for Disease Control in the US has a webpage that lists treatment guidelines for a variety of common medical conditions during pregnancy (https://www.cdc.gov/pregnancy/meds/treatingfortwo/treatment-guidelines.html). Clinics have been developed using a collaborative care model with psychiatrists, social work, and case management integrated within primary care settings, and this approach has been shown to be successful in improving clinical outcomes, secondary prevention of illness, and optimizing care for patients [7]. While caring for the pregnant woman with a psychiatric illness is challenging, it affords an opportunity to intervene in a way that can have a lasting impact for the mother and her baby.

References

1. Abramowitz J, Moore K, Carmin C, Wiegartz PS, Purdon C. Acute onset of obsessive-compulsive disorder in males following childbirth. Psychosomatics. 2001;42(5):429–31. https://doi.org/10.1176/appi.psy.42.5.429.
2. Abramowitz JS, Schwartz SA, Moore KM, Luenzmann KR. Obsessive-compulsive symptoms in pregnancy and the puerperium. J Anxiety Disord. 2003;17:461–78.
3. Abramowitz JS, Khandker M, Nelson CA, Deacon BJ, Rygwall R. The role of cognitive factors in the pathogenesis of obsessive–compulsive symptoms: a prospective study. Behav Res Ther. 2006;44(9):1361–74. https://doi.org/10.1016/j.brat.2005.09.011.
4. American Psychiatric Association. Diagnostic and statistical manual of mental disorders: DSM-5™. 5th ed. (2013-14907-000). Arlington, VA: American Psychiatric Publishing, Inc.; 2013. https://doi.org/10.1176/appi.books.9780890425596.
5. Anda D, Darroch P, Davidson M, Gilly J, Javidi M, Jefford S, Komorowski R, Morejon-Schrobsdorf A. Stress and coping among pregnant adolescents. J Adolesc Res. 1992;7(1):94–109. https://doi.org/10.1177/074355489271007.
6. Anke TMS, Slinning K, Moe V, Brunborg C, Siqveland TS, Skjelstad DV. Mothers with and without bipolar disorder and their infants: group differences in mother-infant interaction patterns at three months postpartum. BMC Psychiatry. 2019;19(1):292. https://doi.org/10.1186/s12888-019-2275-4.
7. Archer J, Bower P, Gilbody S, Lovell K, Richards D, Gask L, Dickens C, Coventry P. Collaborative care for depression and anxiety problems. Cochrane Database Syst Rev. 2012;10:CD006525. https://doi.org/10.1002/14651858.CD006525.pub2. PMID: 23076925.
8. Arnold LM. A case series of women with postpartum-onset obsessive-compulsive disorder. Prim Care Companion J Clin Psychiatry. 1999;1(4):103–8. https://doi.org/10.4088/pcc.v01n0402.
9. Arteche A, Joormann J, Harvey A, Craske M, Gotlib IH, Lehtonen A, Counsell N, Stein A. The effects of postnatal maternal depression and anxiety on the processing of infant faces. J Affect Disord. 2011;133(1–2):197–203. https://doi.org/10.1016/j.jad.2011.04.015.
10. Avenevoli S, Swendsen J, He J-P, Burstein M, Merikangas KR. Major depression in the national comorbidity survey-adolescent supplement: prevalence, correlates, and treatment. J Am Acad Child Adolesc Psychiatry. 2015;54(1):37–44.e2. https://doi.org/10.1016/j.jaac.2014.10.010.

11. Ayers S, Jessop D, Pike A, Parfitt Y, Ford E. The role of adult attachment style, birth intervention and support in posttraumatic stress after childbirth: A prospective study. J Affect Disord. 2014;155:295–8. https://doi.org/10.1016/j.jad.2013.10.022.
12. Barnet B, Joffe A, Duggan AK, Wilson MD, Repke JT. Depressive symptoms, stress, and social support in pregnant and postpartum adolescents. Arch Pediatr Adolesc Med. 1996;150(1):64–9. https://doi.org/10.1001/archpedi.1996.02170260068011.
13. Bauman BL, Ko JY, Cox S, D'Angelo Mph DV, Warner L, Folger S, Tevendale HD, Coy KC, Harrison L, Barfield WD. Vital signs: postpartum depressive symptoms and provider discussions about perinatal depression—United States, 2018. MMWR Morb Mortal Wkly Rep. 2020;69(19):575–81. https://doi.org/10.15585/mmwr.mm6919a2.
14. Behrendt HF, Konrad K, Goecke TW, Fakhrabadi R, Herpertz-Dahlmann B, Firk C. Postnatal mother-to-infant attachment in subclinically depressed mothers: dyads at risk? Psychopathology. 2016;49(4):269–76. https://doi.org/10.1159/000447597.
15. Birmaher B, Axelson D, Strober M, Gill MK, Valeri S, Chiappetta L, Ryan N, Leonard H, Hunt J, Iyengar S, Keller M. Clinical course of children and adolescents with bipolar spectrum disorders. Arch Gen Psychiatry. 2006;63(2):175–83. https://doi.org/10.1001/archpsyc.63.2.175.
16. Bovin MJ, Marx BP, Weathers FW, Gallagher MW, Rodriguez P, Schnurr PP, Keane TM. Psychometric properties of the PTSD checklist for diagnostic and statistical manual of mental disorders-fifth edition (PCL-5) in veterans. Psychol Assess. 2016;28(11):1379–91. https://doi.org/10.1037/pas0000254.
17. Brander G, Rydell M, Kuja-Halkola R, Fernandez de la Cruz L, Lichtenstein P, Serlachius E, Ruck C, Almqvist C, D'Onofrio BM, Larsson H, Mataix-Cols D. Association of perinatal risk factors with obsessive-compulsive disorder: a population-based birth cohort, sibling control study. JAMA Psychiatry. 2016;73(11):1135–44. https://doi.org/10.1001/jamapsychiatry.2016.2095.
18. Challacombe FL, Wroe AL. A hidden problem: consequences of the misdiagnosis of perinatal obsessive-compulsive disorder. Br J Gen Pract. 2013;63(610):275–6. https://doi.org/10.3399/bjgp13X667376.
19. Chan LF, Mohamad Adam B, Norazlin KN, Siti Haida MI, Lee VY, Norazura AW, Ek Zakuan K, Tan SM. Suicidal ideation among single, pregnant adolescents: the role of sexual and religious knowledge, attitudes and practices. J Adolesc. 2016;52:162–9. https://doi.org/10.1016/j.adolescence.2016.08.006. Epub 2016 Aug 27. PMID: 27572955.
20. Christie H, Hamilton-Giachritsis C, Alves-Costa F, Tomlinson M, Halligan SL. The impact of parental posttraumatic stress disorder on parenting: A systematic review. Eur J Psychotraumatol. 2019;10(1):1550345. https://doi.org/10.1080/20008198.2018.1550345.
21. Clout D, Brown R. Sociodemographic, pregnancy, obstetric, and postnatal predictors of postpartum stress, anxiety and depression in new mothers. J Affect Disord. 2015;188:60–7. https://doi.org/10.1016/j.jad.2015.08.054.
22. Coelho FM d C, Pinheiro RT, Silva RA, de Avila Quevedo L, de Mattos Souza LD, de Matos MB, Castelli RD, Pinheiro KAT. Parental bonding and suicidality in pregnant teenagers: A population-based study in southern Brazil. Soc Psychiatry Psychiatr Epidemiol. 2014;49(8):1241–8. https://doi.org/10.1007/s00127-014-0832-1.
23. Creswell C, Apetroaia A, Murray L, Cooper P. Cognitive, affective, and behavioral characteristics of mothers with anxiety disorders in the context of child anxiety disorder. J Abnorm Psychol. 2013;122(1):26–38. https://doi.org/10.1037/a0029516.
24. Das AK, Olfson M, Gameroff MJ, Pilowsky DJ, Blanco C, Feder A, Gross R, Neria Y, Lantigua R, Shea S, Weissman MM. Screening for bipolar disorder in a primary care practice. JAMA. 2005;293(8):956–63. https://doi.org/10.1001/jama.293.8.956.
25. Davidsen KA, Harder S, MacBeth A, Lundy J-M, Gumley A. Mother-infant interaction in schizophrenia: transmitting risk or resilience? A systematic review of the literature. Soc Psychiatry Psychiatr Epidemiol. 2015;50(12):1785–98. https://doi.org/10.1007/s00127-015-1127-x.
26. Dennis C-L, Falah-Hassani K, Brown HK, Vigod SN. Identifying women at risk for postpartum anxiety: a prospective population-based study. Acta Psychiatr Scand. 2016;134(6):485–93. https://doi.org/10.1111/acps.12648.

27. Doghor ON, Nomamiukor FO, Okotcha EN, Onigu-Otite E. Addressing crises in teenage pregnancy. Adolesc Psychiatry. 2019;9(2):69–80. https://doi.org/10.2174/2210676609666190531102808.
28. Eyles DW. How do established developmental risk-factors for schizophrenia change the way the brain develops? Transl Psychiatry. 2021;11(1):158. https://doi.org/10.1038/s41398-021-01273-2.
29. Fairbrother N, Abramowitz JS. New parenthood as a risk factor for the development of obsessional problems. Behav Res Ther. 2007;45(9):2155–63. https://doi.org/10.1016/j.brat.2006.09.019.
30. Fairbrother N, Woody SR. New mothers' thoughts of harm related to the newborn. Arch Womens Ment Health. 2008;11(3):221–9. https://doi.org/10.1007/s00737-008-0016-7.
31. Fairbrother N, Janssen P, Antony MM, Tucker E, Young AH. Perinatal anxiety disorder prevalence and incidence. J Affect Disord. 2016;200:148–55. https://doi.org/10.1016/j.jad.2015.12.082.
32. Feldman R, Granat A, Pariente C, Kanety H, Kuint J, Gilboa-Schechtman E. Maternal depression and anxiety across the postpartum year and infant social engagement, fear regulation, and stress reactivity. J Am Acad Child Adolesc Psychiatry. 2009;48(9):919–27. https://doi.org/10.1097/CHI.0b013e3181b21651.
33. Field T. Prenatal depression effects on early development: a review. Infant Behav Dev. 2011;34(1):1–14. https://doi-org.ezp-prod1.hul.harvard.edu/10.1016/j.infbeh.2010.09.008
34. Field T. Postnatal anxiety prevalence, predictors and effects on development: a narrative review. Infant Behav Dev. 2018;51:24–32. https://doi.org/10.1016/j.infbeh.2018.02.005.
35. Figueiredo B, Pacheco A, Costa R. Depression during pregnancy and the postpartum period in adolescent and adult Portuguese mothers. Arch Womens Ment Health. 2007;10(3):103–9. https://doi.org/10.1007/s00737-007-0178-8.
36. Flaherty LT. Psychoses in adolescents. In: Rosner R, editor. Textbook of adolescent psychiatry. Oxford University Press; 2003. p. 341–5.
37. Fleming N, O'Driscoll T, Becker G, Spitzer RF. Adolescent pregnancy guidelines. J Obstet Gynaecol Can: JOGC (Journal d'obstetrique et Gynecologie Du Canada: JOGC). 2015;37(8):740–56. https://doi.org/10.1016/S1701-2163(15)30180-8.
38. Freitas GV, Cais CF, Stefanello S, Botega NJ. Psychosocial conditions and suicidal behavior in pregnant teenagers: a case-control study in Brazil. Eur Child Adolesc Psychiatry. 2008;17(6):336–42. https://doi.org/10.1007/s00787-007-0668-2. Epub 2008 Apr 21. PMID: 18427870.
39. Gejman PV, Sanders AR, Duan J. The role of genetics in the etiology of schizophrenia. Psychiatr Clin North Am. 2010;33(1):35–66. https://doi.org/10.1016/j.psc.2009.12.003.
40. Gelaye B, Zheng Y, Medina-Mora ME, Rondon MB, Sánchez SE, Williams MA. Validity of the posttraumatic stress disorders (PTSD) checklist in pregnant women. BMC Psychiatry. 2017;17(1):179. https://doi.org/10.1186/s12888-017-1304-4.
41. George A, Luz RF, De Tychey C, Thilly N, Spitz E. Anxiety symptoms and coping strategies in the perinatal period. BMC Pregnancy Childbirth. 2013;13:233. https://doi.org/10.1186/1471-2393-13-233.
42. Goldstein BI, Strober MA, Birmaher B, Axelson DA, Esposito-Smythers C, Goldstein TR, Leonard H, Hunt J, Gill MK, Iyengar S, Grimm C, Yang M, Ryan ND, Keller MB. Substance use disorders among adolescents with bipolar spectrum disorders. Bipolar Disord. 2008;10(4):469–78. https://doi.org/10.1111/j.1399-5618.2008.00584.x.
43. Grekin R, O'Hara MW. Prevalence and risk factors of postpartum posttraumatic stress disorder: A meta-analysis. Clin Psychol Rev. 2014;34(5):389–401. https://doi.org/10.1016/j.cpr.2014.05.003.
44. Heffner JL, DelBello MP, Fleck DE, Adler CM, Strakowski SM. Unplanned pregnancies in adolescents with bipolar disorder. Am J Psychiatr. 2012;169(12):1319. https://doi.org/10.1176/appi.ajp.2012.12060828.
45. Hipwell AE, Murray J, Xiong S, Stepp SD, Keenan KE. Effects of adolescent childbearing on maternal depression and problem behaviors: A prospective, population-based study using

risk-set propensity scores. PLoS One. 2016;11(5):e0155641. https://doi.org/10.1371/journal.pone.0155641.
46. Hodgkinson S, Beers L, Southammakosane C, Lewin A. Addressing the mental health needs of pregnant and parenting adolescents. Pediatrics. 2014;133(1):114–22. https://doi.org/10.1542/peds.2013-0927.
47. House SJ, Tripathi SP, Knight BT, Morris N, Newport DJ, Stowe ZN. Obsessive-compulsive disorder in pregnancy and the postpartum period: course of illness and obstetrical outcome. Arch Womens Ment Health. 2016;19(1):3–10. https://doi.org/10.1007/s00737-015-0542-z.
48. Howard LM, Kumar C, Leese M, Thornicroft G. The general fertility rate in women with psychotic disorders. Am J Psychiatr. 2002;159(6):991–7. https://doi.org/10.1176/appi.ajp.159.6.991.
49. Jellestad L, Vital NA, Malamud J, Taeymans J, Mueller-Pfeiffer C. Functional impairment in posttraumatic stress disorder: a systematic review and meta-analysis. J Psychiatr Res. 2021;136:14–22. https://doi.org/10.1016/j.jpsychires.2021.01.039.
50. Jennings KD, Ross S, Popper S, Elmore M. Thoughts of harming infants in depressed and nondepressed mothers. J Affect Disord. 1999;54(1–2):21–8. https://doi.org/10.1016/s0165-0327(98)00185-2.
51. Johnson KC, Brennan PA, Stowe ZN, Leibenluft E, Newport DJ. Physiological regulation in infants of women with a mood disorder: examining associations with maternal symptoms and stress. J Child Psychol Psychiatry. 2014;55(2):191–8. https://doi.org/10.1111/jcpp.12130.
52. Karukivi M, Tolvanen M, Karlsson H, Karlsson L. Alexithymia and postpartum anxiety and depression symptoms: a follow-up study in a pregnancy cohort. J Psychosom Obstet Gynecol. 2015;36(4):142–7. https://doi.org/10.3109/0167482X.2015.1089228.
53. Kessler M, Ackerson B. Wraparound services: an effective intervention for families impacted by severe mental illness. J Fam Soc Work. 2005;8:29–45. https://doi.org/10.1300/J039v08n04_02.
54. Kessler RC, Berglund PA, Foster CL, Saunders WB, Stang PE, Walters EE. Social consequences of psychiatric disorders, II: teenage parenthood. Am J Psychiatry. 1997;154(10):1405–11. https://doi.org/10.1176/ajp.154.10.1405.
55. Kessler RC, Chiu WT, Demler O, Merikangas KR, Walters EE. Prevalence, severity, and comorbidity of 12-month DSM-IV disorders in the National Comorbidity Survey Replication. Arch Gen Psychiatry. 2005;62(6):617–27. https://doi.org/10.1001/archpsyc.62.6.617.
56. Kessler RC, Avenevoli S, Costello EJ, Georgiades K, Green JG, Gruber MJ, He J, Koretz D, McLaughlin KA, Petukhova M, Sampson NA, Zaslavsky AM, Merikangas KR. Prevalence, persistence, and sociodemographic correlates of DSM-IV disorders in the National Comorbidity Survey Replication Adolescent Supplement. Arch Gen Psychiatry. 2012;69(4):372–80. https://doi.org/10.1001/archgenpsychiatry.2011.160.
57. Kim THM, Connolly JA, Tamim H. The effect of social support around pregnancy on postpartum depression among Canadian teen mothers and adult mothers in the maternity experiences survey. BMC Pregnancy Childbirth. 2014;14:162. https://doi.org/10.1186/1471-2393-14-162.
58. LaRusso EM, Freeman MP. 18—antidepressants in pregnancy. In: Mattison DR, editor. Clinical pharmacology during pregnancy. Academic Press; 2013. p. 295–305. https://doi.org/10.1016/B978-0-12-386007-1.00018-0.
59. Leverich GS, Post RM, Keck PEJ, Altshuler LL, Frye MA, Kupka RW, Nolen WA, Suppes T, McElroy SL, Grunze H, Denicoff K, Moravec MKM, Luckenbaugh D. The poor prognosis of childhood-onset bipolar disorder. J Pediatr. 2007;150(5):485–90. https://doi.org/10.1016/j.jpeds.2006.10.070.
60. Longmore MA, Manning WD, Giordano PC, Rudolph JL. Self-esteem, depressive symptoms, and adolescents' sexual onset. Soc Psychol Q. 2004;67(3):279–95. https://doi.org/10.1177/019027250406700304.
61. Lovejoy MC, Graczyk PA, O'Hare E, Neuman G. Maternal depression and parenting behavior: a meta-analytic review. Clin Psychol Rev. 2000;20(5):561–92. https://doi.org/10.1016/s0272-7358(98)00100-7. PMID: 10860167.
62. Martini J, Petzoldt J, Einsle F, Beesdo-Baum K, Hofler M, Wittchen H-U. Risk factors and course patterns of anxiety and depressive disorders during pregnancy and after delivery: a

prospective-longitudinal study. J Affect Disord. 2015;175:385–95. https://doi.org/10.1016/j.jad.2015.01.012.
63. Milan S, Ickovics JR, Kershaw T, Lewis J, Meade C, Ethier K. Prevalence, course, and predictors of emotional distress in pregnant and parenting adolescents. J Consult Clin Psychol. 2004;72(2):328–40. https://doi.org/10.1037/0022-006X.72.2.328.
64. Miller ES, Hoxha D, Wisner KL, Gossett DR. Obsessions and compulsions in postpartum women without obsessive compulsive disorder. J Womens Health (Larchmt). 2015;24(10):825–30. https://doi.org/10.1089/jwh.2014.5063.
65. Miron O, Yu K-H, Wilf-Miron R, Kohane IS. Suicide rates among adolescents and young adults in the United States, 2000–2017. JAMA. 2019;321(23):2362–4. https://doi.org/10.1001/jama.2019.5054.
66. Misri SK. Obsessive-compulsive disorders in new fathers: feeling out of control. In: Misri SK, editor. Paternal postnatal psychiatric illnesses: a clinical case book. Cham: Springer; 2018. p. 81–99.
67. Mitsuhiro SS, Chalem E, Moraes Barros MC, Guinsburg R, Laranjeira R. Brief report: prevalence of psychiatric disorders in pregnant teenagers. J Adolesc. 2009;32(3):747–52. https://doi.org/10.1016/j.adolescence.2008.12.001.
68. Mohamadirizi S, Kordi M, Shakeri MT, Modares-Gharavi M. The relationship between eating disorder symptoms and obsessive compulsive disorder in primigravida women. Iran J Nurs Midwifery Res. 2015;20(6):642–6. https://doi.org/10.4103/1735-9066.170015.
69. Mojtabai R, Olfson M, Han B. National trends in the prevalence and treatment of depression in adolescents and young adults. Pediatrics. 2016;138(6) https://doi.org/10.1542/peds.2016-1878.
70. Mollborn S, Morningstar E. Investigating the relationship between teenage childbearing and psychological distress using longitudinal evidence. J Health Soc Behav. 2009;50(3):310–26. https://doi.org/10.1177/002214650905000305.
71. Muzik M, Borovska S. Perinatal depression: implications for child mental health. Ment Health Fam Med. 2010;7(4):239–47.
72. Namouz-Haddad S, Nulman I. Safety of treatment of obsessive compulsive disorder in pregnancy and puerperium. Can Fam Physician. 2014;60(2):133–6.
73. Nicol-Harper R, Harvey AG, Stein A. Interactions between mothers and infants: impact of maternal anxiety. Infant Behav Dev. 2007;30(1):161–7. https://doi.org/10.1016/j.infbeh.2006.08.005.
74. Nillni YI, Mehralizade A, Mayer L, Milanovic S. Treatment of depression, anxiety, and trauma-related disorders during the perinatal period: A systematic review. Clin Psychol Rev. 2018;66:136–48. https://doi-org.ezp-prod1.hul.harvard.edu/10.1016/j.cpr.2018.06.004
75. Ornoy A, Weinstein-Fudim L, Ergaz Z. Antidepressants, antipsychotics, and mood stabilizers in pregnancy: what do we know and how should we treat pregnant women with depression. Birth Defects Res. 2017;109(12):933–56. https://doi.org/10.1002/bdr2.1079. PMID: 28714604.
76. Orsolini L, Valchera A, Vecchiotti R, Tomasetti C, Iasevoli F, Fornaro M, De Berardis D, Perna G, Pompili M, Bellantuono C. Suicide during perinatal period: epidemiology, risk factors, and clinical correlates. Front Psychiatry. 2016;7:138. https://doi.org/10.3389/fpsyt.2016.00138. PMID: 27570512; PMCID: PMC4981602.
77. Owen MJ, Sawa A, Mortensen PB. Schizophrenia. Lancet (London, England). 2016;388(10039):86–97. https://doi.org/10.1016/S0140-6736(15)01121-6.
78. Prins A, Ouimette P, Kimerling R, Cameron RP, Hugelshofer DS, Shaw-Hegwer J, Thrailkill A, Gusman FD, Sheikh JI. The primary care PTSD screen (PC-PTSD): development and operating characteristics. Prim Care Psychiatry. 2003;9:9–14. https://doi.org/10.1185/135525703125002360. PTSDpubs ID: 26676
79. Radke-Yarrow M, Cummings EM, Kuczynski L, Chapman M. Patterns of attachment in two- and three-year-olds in normal families and families with parental depression. Child Dev. 1985;56(4):884–93. PMID: 4042751.

80. Ramsauer B, Achtergarde S. Mothers with acute and chronic postpartum psychoses and impact on the mother-infant interaction. Schizophr Res. 2018;197:45–58. https://doi.org/10.1016/j.schres.2018.02.032.
81. Reid V, Meadows-Oliver M. Postpartum depression in adolescent mothers: an integrative review of the literature. J Pediatr Health Care. 2007;21(5):289–98. https://doi.org/10.1016/j.pedhc.2006.05.010.
82. Rodriguez MR, Nuevo R, Chatterji S, Ayuso-Mateos JL. Definitions and factors associated with subthreshold depressive conditions: a systematic review. BMC Psychiatry. 2012;12:181. https://doi.org/10.1186/1471-244X-12-181.
83. Ruscio AM, Stein DJ, Chiu WT, Kessler RC. The epidemiology of obsessive-compulsive disorder in the National Comorbidity Survey Replication. Mol Psychiatry. 2010;15(1):53–63. https://doi.org/10.1038/mp.2008.94.
84. Rusner M, Berg M, Begley C. Bipolar disorder in pregnancy and childbirth: a systematic review of outcomes. BMC Pregnancy Childbirth. 2016;16(1):331. https://doi.org/10.1186/s12884-016-1127-1.
85. Russell EJ, Fawcett JM, Mazmanian D. Risk of obsessive-compulsive disorder in pregnant and postpartum women: a meta-analysis. J Clin Psychiatry. 2013;74(4):377–85. https://doi.org/10.4088/JCP.12r07917.
86. Schmidt RM, Wiemann CM, Rickert VI, Smith EO. Moderate to severe depressive symptoms among adolescent mothers followed four years postpartum. J Adolesc Health. 2006;38(6):712–8. https://doi.org/10.1016/j.jadohealth.2005.05.023. PMID: 16730600.
87. Seng JS, Low LK, Sperlich M, Ronis DL, Liberzon I. Prevalence, trauma history, and risk for posttraumatic stress disorder among nulliparous women in maternity care. Obstet Gynecol. 2009;114(4):839–47. https://doi.org/10.1097/AOG.0b013e3181b8f8a2.
88. Shalev A, Liberzon I, Marmar C. Post-traumatic stress disorder. N Engl J Med. 2017;376(25):2459–69. https://doi.org/10.1056/NEJMra1612499.
89. Siegel RS, Brandon AR. Adolescents, pregnancy, and mental health. J Pediatr Adolesc Gynecol. 2014;27(3):138–50. https://doi.org/10.1016/j.jpag.2013.09.008.
90. Sit D. Women and bipolar disorder across the life span. J Am Med Womens Assoc (1972). 2004;59(2):91–100.
91. Spiegel DR, Sommese K, Turenkov A, Naimon N. A case of peripartum obsessive-compulsive disorder: the potential role of corticosteroids, gonadal steroids, and the neuropeptide oxytocin in its pathogenesis. Innov Clin Neurosci. 2019;16(5–6):41–5.
92. Strand J, Boström P, Grip K. Parents' descriptions of how their psychosis affects parenting. J Child Fam Stud. 2020;29:620–31. https://doi.org/10.1007/s10826-019-01605-3.
93. Substance Abuse and Mental Health Services Administration Trauma-informed care in behavioral health services. Treatment improvement protocol (TIP) series 57. HHS Publication No. (SMA) 13-4801. Rockville, MD: Substance Abuse and Mental Health Services Administration; 2014. https://www.ncbi.nlm.nih.gov/books/NBK207201/pdf/Bookshelf_NBK207201.pdf.
94. Tabet M, Flick LH, Cook CAL, Xian H, Chang JJ. Age at first birth and psychiatric disorders in low-income pregnant women. J Womens Health (Larchmt). 2016;25(8):810–7. https://doi.org/10.1089/jwh.2015.5236.
95. Thiel F, Eberhard-Gran M, Garthus-Niegel S. The impact of perinatal life stress on infant temperament and child development: A 2-year follow-up cohort study. J Dev Behav Pediatr: JDBP. 2020;42:299. https://doi.org/10.1097/DBP.0000000000000887.
96. Tietz A, Zietlow A-L, Reck C. Maternal bonding in mothers with postpartum anxiety disorder: the crucial role of subclinical depressive symptoms and maternal avoidance behaviour. Arch Women Ment Health. 2014;17(5):433–42. https://doi.org/10.1007/s00737-014-0423-x.
97. Troutman BR, Cutrona CE. Nonpsychotic postpartum depression among adolescent mothers. J Abnorm Psychol. 1990;99(1):69–78. https://doi.org/10.1037/0021-843X.99.1.69.
98. Twenge JM, Cooper AB, Joiner TE, Duffy ME, Binau SG. Age, period, and cohort trends in mood disorder indicators and suicide-related outcomes in a nationally representative dataset, 2005–2017. J Abnorm Psychol. 2019;128(3):185–99. https://doi.org/10.1037/abn0000410.

99. Uguz F. Pharmacotherapy of obsessive-compulsive disorder during pregnancy: A clinical approach. Rev Bras Psiquiatr (Sao Paulo, Brazil: 1999). 2015;37(4):334–42. https://doi.org/10.1590/1516-4446-2015-1673.
100. Uguz F, Gezginc K, Zeytinci IE, Karatayli S, Askin R, Guler O, Kir Sahin F, Emul HM, Ozbulut O, Gecici O. Obsessive-compulsive disorder in pregnant women during the third trimester of pregnancy. Compr Psychiatry. 2007;48(5):441–5. https://doi.org/10.1016/j.comppsych.2007.05.001.
101. van Os J, Kapur S. Schizophrenia. Lancet. 2009;374(9690):635–45. https://doi.org/10.1016/S0140-6736(09)60995-8.
102. Vigod SN, Dennis CL, Kurdyak PA, Cairney J, Guttmann A, Taylor VH. Fertility rate trends among adolescent girls with major mental illness: A population-based study. Pediatrics. 2014;133(3):e585–91. https://doi.org/10.1542/peds.2013-1761.
103. Viswasam K, Eslick GD, Starcevic V. Prevalence, onset and course of anxiety disorders during pregnancy: A systematic review and meta analysis. J Affect Disord. 2019;255:27–40. https://doi.org/10.1016/j.jad.2019.05.016.
104. Wagner KD, Hirschfeld RM, Emslie GJ, Findling RL, Gracious BL, Reed ML. Validation of the mood disorder questionnaire for bipolar disorders in adolescents. J Clin Psychiatry. 2006;67(5):827–30. https://doi-org.ezp-prod1.hul.harvard.edu/10.4088/jcp.v67n0518
105. Zambaldi CF, Cantilino A, Montenegro AC, Paes JA, de Albuquerque TLC, Sougey EB. Postpartum obsessive-compulsive disorder: prevalence and clinical characteristics. Compr Psychiatry. 2009;50(6):503–9. https://doi.org/10.1016/j.comppsych.2008.11.014.
106. Zhang T, Zhao B, Shi C, Nie B, Liu H, Yang X, Sun Y, Li P, Lin L, Yang X, Li J, Gao X, Feng S, Li X, Sun X, Pan T, Feng T, Bao T, Shan B. Subthreshold depression may exist on a spectrum with major depressive disorder: evidence from gray matter volume and morphological brain network. J Affect Disord. 2020;266:243–51. https://doi.org/10.1016/j.jad.2020.01.135.
107. Zipursky RB, Reilly TJ, Murray RM. The myth of schizophrenia as a progressive brain disease. Schizophr Bull. 2013;39(6):1363–72. https://doi.org/10.1093/schbul/sbs135.

Substance Use

9

Lois T. Flaherty

The prevalence of illicit drug use among pregnant women is highest among adolescents and young adults. The 2016 National Survey on Drug Use and Health reported past-month illicit drug use rates among pregnant women of 14.3% for those aged 15–17, 10.1% among those aged 18–25, compared to 5.6% among women aged 26–44 years. Nicotine is the most used substance among pregnant teens, followed by alcohol, cannabis, and other illicit substances [69].

Substance use refers to the use of alcohol, tobacco, or illicit drugs, including non-medical use of prescription drugs. For persons under 21 in the USA, the term illicit applies to any use of alcohol, cannabis, and nicotine, possession of which is illegal. Substance use disorders involve a pattern of use characterized by tolerance, craving, inability to control use, and continued use despite adverse consequences. A diagnosis is based on specific criteria such as unsuccessful efforts to cut down or control use, as well as use resulting in social problems and a failure to fulfill obligations at work, school, or home [3].

Characteristics

The US Substance Abuse and Mental Health Services Administration, which does periodic surveys of representative samples of the US population, reported that in 2018, an estimated 164.8 million people aged 12 or older in the USA (60.2%) had used one or more illicit substances in the past month (2019). Recent data show declines in substance abuse among all teenagers [78], and pregnant adolescents tend to stop or decrease their use of substances as soon as they find out they are pregnant [72].

Adolescents who use substances are at higher risk for pregnancy than those who do not, with almost 60% of pregnant teens reporting past use—twice the rate of use

L. T. Flaherty (✉)
Harvard Medical School, Cambridge, MA, USA

J.-V. P. Wittenberg et al. (eds.), *Adolescent Pregnancy and Parenting*,
https://doi.org/10.1007/978-3-031-42502-8_9

by non-pregnant teens. These discrepancies hold even when socio-demographic and family factors are controlled for [72]. One possible explanation may be the disinhibition and impairment in judgment associated with many substances. For example, unplanned intercourse under the influence of alcohol or drugs is associated with decreased condom use and multiple partners [68].

Fetal and Infant Consequences

The ability of the abused substance to cross the placental barrier determines the effect it may have on the fetus and has been studied by researchers for virtually all drugs of abuse using animal models. The effects can be severe and permanent, such as in the case of fetal alcohol syndrome. Sithisarn et al. [75] reviewed studies on the effects of specific substances, including nicotine, alcohol, cannabis, cocaine, opiates, and methamphetamine. They found that manifestations of prenatal exposure to these substances included "varying deficits in birth anthropometric measurements, mild-to-moderate transient neurobehavioral alterations in infancy and long-term behavioral problems noted from early childhood to adolescence." They also noted that the severity of expression of behavioral problems was influenced by environmental factors.

Evidence shows that substances of abuse can impede the transfer of nutrients to the fetus. For example, tetrahydrocannabinol, the psychoactive ingredient in cannabis, has been shown in rat models to prevent the placental transfer of glucose, a key nutrient, from the mother to the fetus, and is associated with reduced placental vasculature suggesting reduced blood flow from the mother to the fetus [59].

Overview of Common Substances of Abuse

Nicotine

Although nicotine use has declined among young people, the inhalation of smokeless tobacco from electronic cigarettes, known as vaping, has increased dramatically among teens to the point that it surpasses cigarette smoking [33]. According to the CDC, in 2020, 23.6% of high school students reported current use of a tobacco product [34].

Nicotine, the psychoactive ingredient in tobacco products, is highly addictive. The risk factors for nicotine use among adolescents overlap with risk factors for other kinds of substance use and with risk for pregnancy. These include poor school performance, risk taking, depression, and anxiety [7].

Cornelius et al. [23], studying a cohort of pregnant adolescents between 1990 and 1994 (aged 12–18), found that 52% reported smoking cigarettes in the year prior to pregnancy. Among rural populations, rates are even higher. One study in West Virginia found that 67% of pregnant women under the age of 19 smoked [2].

Data suggest that many teens attempt to stop smoking when they find out they are pregnant, although relapse is common both during and after the pregnancy [21]. Cornelius and colleagues in the study cited above [23] found the rate dropped from 52% prior to the pregnancy to 46% in the first trimester, but then rose to 58% by the third trimester.

Although the number of cigarettes per day smoked by pregnant women tends to be lower among teenagers than older women, teens who smoke during pregnancy are at high risk for becoming addicted later in life [10]. Some pregnant women, including teens, turn to vaping from smoking to discontinue or reduce smoking, and in the belief that vaping is safer than smoking. Vaping, like smoking, delivers nicotine, and although it does not contain the same harmful substances as cigarette smoke, additives in e-cigarettes can be harmful. While research on the effects of vaping on the fetus is limited, there is emerging evidence that like smoking, it may increase the risk of being born small for gestational age [58].

Sales of electronic cigarettes to teens have increasingly been prohibited by states in the USA, with the unintended consequence that more teens have turned to smoking. Pesko and Currie (2019) found that the passage of laws restricting sales of electronic cigarettes to minors was associated with a rise in smoking among pregnant teens.

Effects on Children Nicotine passes through the placenta and is also present in breast milk. Animal studies have shown it affects the developing brain by causing persistent gene alterations in brain regions involved in the reward pathway and neurodevelopmental changes at the cellular level [46]. In addition, it may compromise placental efficiency, leading to reduced nutrient transport and blood flow [51].

Although harmful effects of nicotine on fetuses were known since the 1950s [52, 74], it was not until 1984 that specific warnings about smoking during pregnancy were required on all cigarette packages and advertisements (Comprehensive Smoking Education Act of 1984; Public Law 98–474).

The first observations were that babies born to mothers who smoked during pregnancy tended to be small for gestational age. Since that time many other problems have been well documented. Cornelius and Day [22] summarized these problems as follows.

Prenatal tobacco exposure (PTE) affects speech processing, levels of irritability and hypertonicity, attention levels, ability to self-regulate, need to be handled, and response to novelty preference in infants. In early childhood, PTE effects were mostly behavioral outcomes including activity and inattention and externalizing behaviors, including conduct disorder and antisocial behavior. In adolescents, PTE predicted increased attention-deficit/hyperactivity disorder, modulation of the cerebral cortex and white matter structure, and nicotine addiction (p. 121).

Interventions Smoking cessation is a challenge for all people, including pregnant women. Interventions can be categorized as psychosocial or pharmacological. Generally, psychosocial interventions are preferable since they avoid the risk of pharmacological agents. Behavioral interventions usually involve individual or group counseling, and computer driven interventions have been implemented. Evidence for efficacy for any of these is limited. A Cochrane database report that evaluated psychosocial interventions for young people concluded:

> There is limited evidence that either behavioral support or smoking cessation medication increases the proportion of young people that stop smoking in the long term. Findings are most promising for group-based behavioral interventions, but evidence remains limited for all intervention types [30].

This report, however, excluded studies that focused on pregnant young women. Pregnant adolescents who smoke tend to smoke fewer cigarettes than older women, so smoking cessation might be easier for them, and they may be more able to stop with non-pharmacological interventions, including counseling and education. The most recent Cochrane report specifically focusing on pregnant adolescents and young women did find a moderate degree of efficacy for psychosocial interventions, specifically citing counseling, feedback, and incentives as effective [14]. One example of such a program is the American Lung Association's Not-On-Tobacco (N-O-T) program, designed for 14–19-year-old smokers who want to quit (https://www.lung.org/quit-smoking/smoking-facts/tobacco-use-among-children).

Pharmacological approaches include nicotine replacement therapy (NRT) via patches and chewing gum, and the drugs bupropion (Zyban®) and varenicline (Chantix® or Champix®). These treatments have been shown to work in non-pregnant smokers, but data on the use of these in pregnant women have been limited and mostly derived from small non-randomized studies. A Cochrane database review published in 2020 concluded there was no evidence supporting either positive or negative effects of NRT on birth outcomes [17]. This review also found that efficacy of bupropion based on randomized placebo-controlled trials was lacking. They cited an absence of randomized controlled trials for either varenicline or electronic cigarettes.

Treatment with nicotine delivery systems has generally been recommended as safer than the other pharmacological treatments. These deliver nicotine in a more gradual way than smoking or vaping and do not produce a "high," so they eliminate withdrawal as a component of addiction. Although transdermal and oral preparations deliver nicotine to the fetus, they do not contain the harmful ingredients of smoke or e-cigarettes. However, a recently published large scale population-based cohort study of women who smoked during pregnancy indicated that the rate of adverse birth outcomes was not increased among women who used any of these pharmacological treatments compared with those who did not, and varenicline was actually associated with lower rates of adverse outcomes [83]. Given the known harmful effects of smoking on the fetus, and the difficulty pregnant women have in stopping, the use of such delivery methods seems to entail a reasonable risk–benefit ratio.

At this time there is some evidence e-cigarettes are marginally less harmful than smoked cigarettes, and that switching from smoking to vaping may reduce harm

[58], but vaping is hardly to be encouraged and all major guidelines strongly advise against it. Bupropion and varenicline do not appear to be harmful during pregnancy; a meta-analysis concluded there was no strong evidence that either major positive or negative fetal outcomes were associated with gestational use of bupropion or varenicline [84].

Bupropion is an antidepressant, but its antismoking effects seem to be separate from the antidepressant effects. The mechanism of the antismoking activity of bupropion is not fully understood but is thought to be related to blocking the symptoms of nicotine withdrawal by inhibiting reuptake of dopamine, noradrenaline, and serotonin in the central nervous system [70]. Varenicline is a nicotine receptor partial agonist, thus it partly stimulates nicotine receptors, mimicking the effects of nicotine and reducing cravings and withdrawal symptoms. At the same time, it partially blocks nicotine receptors, preventing nicotine from attaching to them and blocking the effects of exogenous nicotine.

In summary, tobacco use is a major public health problem and one that is relatively refractory to treatment. Although nicotine addiction is not a commonly used term to apply to the use of tobacco products, the highly addictive nature of nicotine places it in a similar category to alcohol, opiates, and stimulants. Like alcohol it is legally available and even though sales to minors are illegal, it is easily obtainable by adolescents. We are still dealing with depictions of cigarette smoking as a pleasurable, socially acceptable activity and more recently, the marketing of e-cigarettes to young people. It is inevitable that many young women who smoke or vape will become pregnant. Most of these young women will want to discontinue using tobacco and many will be able to do so with the help and support of health care providers. It seems intuitive that a combination of psychosocial and pharmacological interventions will have the best chance of success.

Alcohol

Alcohol is one of the most widely used and misused substances worldwide and is the most used illicit substance by teens in the USA [57]. It is also the second most used substance by pregnant teens [69].

Binge drinking is the most common form of alcohol consumption among teenagers and transition age youth [72]. Binge drinking is defined as the amount that typically produces blood alcohol levels of ≥0.08% [61]. Typically, this is five drinks consumed over 2 h by adult males and four drinks by adult females, but for young adolescents, the threshold of what constitutes binge drinking can be as low as three drinks. Binge drinking is associated with high risk sexual activity, and thus increases risk of unplanned pregnancy. When they drink, young people become less concerned with risks, less discriminating regarding sexual partners, and less likely to insist on safer sex practices. In fact, some drink to reduce inhibitions about sexual activity [12].

Salas-Wright and colleagues found in a study that used data from the National Survey on Drug Use and Health between 2002 and 2012 (n = 97,850), that about

1 in 6 pregnant teens reported using alcohol within 30 days of being surveyed (15.85%). However, reported use was highest among teens in their first trimester and was much less among those in the second and third trimesters. Their findings, albeit cross-sectional, did suggest teens decreased their use markedly over the course of the pregnancy, but much of their drinking occurred before they knew they were pregnant, when it is likely to have had maximal deleterious effects.

Effects on Children Concerns about alcohol use during pregnancy surfaced in the 1970s when fetal alcohol syndrome (FAS) was recognized [43]. Of all the consequences of substance use during pregnancy this is the most serious, causing severe and lifelong effects. Signs of FAS include growth impairment, dysmorphic facial features (short palpebral fissures, smooth or flattened philtrum, thin upper lip), and central nervous system abnormalities, including microcephaly [90, p.18]. Fetal alcohol spectrum disorders comprise a continuum from mild to severe, with neurodevelopmental problems being common to all. Learning disabilities are common and have their own long-term consequences, among them academic failure, substance abuse, mental health problems, contact with law enforcement, and an inability to live independently and obtain and maintain employment.

In addition to FAS, maternal alcohol use has been associated with lower birth weight and gestational age, and with aggressive and delinquent behavior as well as anxious and depressed and withdrawn behavior in children as measured by both internalizing and externalizing behavior [77].

The etiology of FAS is complex, with alcohol being the major, but not the only, factor involved. Patterns of drinking (binge drinking) and timing (first trimester) are important, as are concomitant smoking and poor diet. However, as Abel has pointed out, FAS is "not an equal opportunity birth defect" [1]. The harmful effects of alcohol on the fetus are mediated by and have long been known to disproportionately affect poor and minority populations [1, 8]. For example, more than 30 years ago it was estimated that in the Yukon and Northwest areas of Canada native children were 1000 times more likely than non-native children to have FAS—rates of FAS were estimated to be 46/1000 for Native children compared to 0.4/1000 for non-Native children [4]. While not quite as horrifying, figures for the USA are also startling, with the rate of FAS among low-income populations ten times greater than that of middle- and high-income populations—2.29/1000 compared to 0.26/1000 [1].

While some of the early studies have been criticized as having methodological deficiencies, more recent comprehensive reviews have confirmed that there are major disparities among subpopulations worldwide, with poverty and minority status being key risk factors [53, 55]. Popova and colleagues, based on a meta-analysis of the literature, estimated the global prevalence of FAS in the general population to be 14.6 per 10,000, with a pregnant woman's risk of having a child with FAS if she drinks during the pregnancy at 1 in 67 [67].

The fact that most women, including teens, reduce or stop their alcohol intake when they plan to become pregnant or discover they are pregnant suggests that most of them do not have an addiction to alcohol. However, it does exist.

Current clinical guidelines recommend inquiring about alcohol use during initial and subsequent antenatal visits and referring for treatment if required, as well as educating patients about the risks of consumption during pregnancy and recommending that they not use alcohol at all while they are pregnant [9, 31]. This is not universally done [25], indicating that steps need to be taken to improve health care providers' adherence to these guidelines.

Brief questionnaires have been shown to be useful for screening. The 9 question CRAFFT screens for both alcohol and substance use. The CRAFFT is freely available as a clinician administered as well as self-report questionnaire (www.ceasar.org).

Cannabis

After alcohol, cannabis is the most widely used illicit substance worldwide (WHO), as well as among US adolescents (MTF) and pregnant women [86]. It is available in many forms and can be inhaled or eaten. The cannabis available for recreational use has become stronger over the years, meaning that the potential for adverse side effects has steadily increased. Recent trends in the USA and Canada of legalization of recreational and medical cannabis have sparked concerns about the use of cannabinoids by pregnant women [40].

Volkow and colleagues, in a study of marijuana use among pregnant women in the USA, found rates highest among those 25 and younger, as well as among non-Hispanic Black women. Strikingly, although in general pregnant women used less than non-pregnant women, pregnant adolescents (aged 12–17) had higher rates of use than non-pregnant teens [86], with 14% of pregnant teens reporting past month use, compared to 6% of non-pregnant girls.

A study published in 2015 found 18% of pregnant women who used marijuana were dependent and/or misusing it [48].

Studies have shown that some pregnant women are using cannabis to relieve nausea and stress, with the belief that as a natural substance it is less harmful than prescription drugs [6]. This trend prompted the USA Surgeon General to issue an advisory that warned women not to use marijuana to alleviate nausea during pregnancy [60].

Effects on Children A mother's cannabis use during pregnancy may increase the risk of low birth weight and small for gestational age births, preterm births, and may also increase the risk of neonatal intensive care unit placement and developmental problems [36, 47].

THC has been shown to cross the placenta in animal models, with fetal plasma levels increasing with repetitive exposure. In addition, research on rat models have shown that THC reduces blood flow to the fetus and prevents oxygen and nutrients from crossing the placenta into the developing fetus, while studies of human placental cells have indicated that THC prevents placental transfer of glucose by decreasing a glucose transporter GLUT-1 [59]. THC has also been found in human breast milk [65].

There are a considerable number of studies implicating prenatal cannabis exposure with later behavior problems, including adolescent cannabis use. Prenatal cannabis exposure may affect cognitive development by increasing the risk of hyperactivity, impulsivity, and inability to focus [24, 42]. It also predisposes offspring to neuropsychiatric disorders [64]. A recent systematic review linked prenatal exposure to later affective symptoms and ADHD [71]. Second-hand cannabis use may present issues in pregnancy, as researchers at Boston University found cannabis use among men may double the risk of partner miscarriage—regardless of the woman's use [39].

Some of the effects of cannabis on fetal development may be due to toxic effects of smoke, like those of tobacco smoke. Furthermore, cannabis use is more likely in low income, socially disadvantaged young women and the supposed effects may in fact be due to other risk factors among teens who misuse substances and become pregnant, such as poor nutrition, lack of prenatal care, and so on [50, 89].

Nevertheless, the data are concerning. The American College of Obstetrics and Gynecology (ACOG) felt that the evidence was sufficiently compelling to recommend against any use of cannabis during pregnancy or lactation [20]. They cited studies showing evidence of cognitive impairment, including visual problem solving, visual–motor coordination, visual analysis, attention, poorer reading and spelling scores and lower teacher-perceived school performance.

The ACOG report noted the importance of endocannabinoids and endocannabinoid receptors in the brain during fetal development, with the implication that exogenous cannabinoids in the form of marijuana might interfere with these essential processes in brain development. It has been suggested that this interference could affect the prefrontal cortex, the mesolimbic system, the striatum, and the hypothalamic-pituitary axis, which are involved in executive functions and the reinforcement and regulation of the emotional systems [71].

ACOG guidelines call for educating women about the effects of cannabis and discouraging use, including the use of cannabis for medicinal purposes [20]. Cannabis use can be addictive for some. Psychosocial interventions are similar as for other forms of substance abuse [35]. Although some pharmacologic interventions appear promising, overall, there is insufficient evidence for efficacy and there are no data on safety and efficacy in pregnancy [49].

Stimulants

Stimulants include cocaine, methamphetamines, ecstasy (MDMA), and various prescription stimulant drugs, such as methylphenidate, dextroamphetamine, and derivatives. Use of cocaine is highest among the young adult age group (18–25), while methamphetamine use is most prevalent in adults aged 26–49 [79]. As a group, these are the second most abused substances during pregnancy [76]. These drugs all act on the brain dopamine system and have a high abuse potential, as well as causing behavioral and cognitive impairments. Psychological effects of stimulant use include decreased sexual inhibitions; use during adolescence is associated with risky sexual behavior and adolescent pregnancy [29, 92]. Furthermore, there are shared risk factors for pregnancy and methamphetamine use. These include depression, low self-esteem, and sensation-seeking behavior [92].

Stimulants have become a major cause of deaths due to overdose; overall, stimulant-related deaths in 2018 accounted for roughly 40% of all overdose deaths in the USA [13].

Methamphetamine

Among stimulants, methamphetamine has been cited as particularly dangerous and has become a major concern in the USA as well as worldwide, where use ranks just below cannabis. Although in general adolescents are less likely than adults to use this drug, use among this group has been increasing. A study of admissions to federally funded treatment centers in the USA using data that tracked admissions from 1994 to 2006 found that the percentage of admissions for methamphetamine treatment among pregnant women rose from 8% to 24% over that period, making it the primary substance compelling treatment during pregnancy.

Effects on Children Two systematic reviews of research on consequences of the use of methamphetamine during pregnancy concluded that there are adverse effects of the fetus—low gestational age, low birth weight, and decreased head circumference and body length, but no significant effects on pregnancy complications, such as hypertension [45, 91]. The Wright study controlled for possible confounding factors, including tobacco use, poverty, poor diet, and lack of prenatal care.

Methamphetamine use by parents is well known to be associated with severe abuse and neglect and children of active users are usually placed in foster care [54]. In addition to physical and psychological harm experienced by children, hyperactivity, and externalizing behavior problems are common [26].

Interventions Treatment for methamphetamine use disorders and problematic methamphetamine use is challenging. A report by the Canadian Agency for Drugs and Technologies in Health found "no evidence-based guidelines were identified regarding withdrawal management or long-term treatment for persons who are pregnant and addicted to crystal methamphetamine" [16]. Another recent review noted there is "no clear best approach" [38].

Chan et al. [15] reviewed the evidence for efficacy of pharmacologic approaches and found the only agent for which there was any evidence was methylphenidate, and even for this the quality of evidence was low. They noted dopamine agonists, GABA agents, antipsychotics, and antidepressants have been tried but evidence for efficacy is lacking.

Opioids

Opioid use during pregnancy includes both prescription and non-prescription drug use. Most commonly it involves heroin, codeine, oxycodone (Oxycontin), methadone, or buprenorphine. Opioid use disorders (OUDs) among pregnant women have been increasing rapidly [81].

Opioid use during pregnancy is often associated with other psychiatric comorbidity, especially depression [28, 41]. As is the case for the general population, chronic pain is a significant risk factor [28].

Effects on Children The major danger with prenatal opioid use is neonatal abstinence syndrome, in which the infant is born addicted to a drug and goes through a variety of withdrawal symptoms. These can include tremors, jitteriness, hyperirritability, excessive crying, and diarrhea, and rarely, seizures.

Interventions Medication-assisted treatment (MAT) is the standard of care for opioid dependence and addiction. This usually involves either methadone or buprenorphine, as part of a comprehensive treatment program that includes psychosocial interventions. Until 2010, methadone was the standard of care for treatment of opioid addiction during pregnancy. However, methadone can only be given in special opioid treatment programs, limiting access to treatment. Buprenorphine has the advantage that it can be given in office-based practices by physicians who are trained and certified in its use, including obstetricians. Buprenorphine, a partial Mu agonist, in contrast with methadone, which is a full Mu agonist, is associated with less severe neonatal abstinence syndrome. Several studies have found buprenorphine to be as good or better than methadone, beginning with a double blinded multi-site, multi-national study [44]. This study involved a total of 175 women, some as young as 18, all of whom received comprehensive care. Babies born to the mothers on buprenorphine required less morphine for the treatment of NAS, experienced shorter duration of treatment for NAS, and shorter hospital stays than did infants with prenatal exposure to methadone [44]. This study did, however, have a higher dropout rate for the buprenorphine group (33% vs. 18%), the reasons for which were unclear.

Meyer and colleagues retrospectively compared methadone and buprenorphine outcomes in a cohort of over 600 opioid-dependent pregnant women, looking at maternal characteristics, prenatal care, and newborn outcomes. They found better outcomes in the buprenorphine treated group, with mothers treated with buprenorphine more likely to start medication before or earlier in pregnancy. Their infants were less likely to be premature or have low birth weights, as well as less likely to require treatment for neonatal abstinence [56].

Naltrexone, an opioid antagonist, has been used to treat alcohol use disorders for many years and has demonstrated safety. It is also used to treat opioid addiction in pregnant women and appears to be safe in this population but data on efficacy are limited. Since it is not an opioid agonist, there is a requirement of 7–10 days of medically supervised withdrawal from opioids before starting naltrexone, raising concerns about relapse. A recent study, however, demonstrated that there was not a significant amount of relapse, the risk of NAS was markedly reduced, and the drug appeared to be safe and effective [82]. It is an alternative for women who wish to eliminate opioid use entirely.

Hallucinogens

Hallucinogenic drugs include lysergic acid diethylamide (LSD), phencyclidine (PCP), peyote, mescaline, psilocybin mushrooms, "Ecstasy" (MDMA or "Molly"), ketamine, DMT/AMT/"Foxy," and salvia divinorum. In recent years there has been a resurgence of interest in possible medical applications of LSD and a concomitant concern about renewed popularity of recreational use. The most recent figures available indicate the use of hallucinogens by adolescents aged 12–17 is relatively infrequent compared to other illicit drugs (1.5%), and hallucinogen use has been decreasing among this group. However, the rate of hallucinogen use is 6.9% for older adolescents and young adults aged 18–25 [78]. As of this writing there are no published epidemiological studies of the prevalence of hallucinogen use by pregnant women of any age, but given the existing data on use among teenagers and young adults, and the likelihood of pregnancy among this age group, some use among young pregnant women is inevitable.

Nichols and Grob [63], in a review of published literature related to LSD toxicity, concluded that LSD has a very low toxicity, with most of the deaths attributed to the drug being caused by other factors, such as dangerous behavior under the influence of the drug or the imposition of physical restraints resulting in asphyxia. However, long-term effects of hallucinogens include persistent psychosis, visual disturbances, disorganized thinking, paranoia, mood disturbances, hallucinogen persisting perception disorder, hallucinations, and other visual disturbances (such as seeing halos or trails attached to moving objects). Tolerance does develop with some drugs but disappears a few days after cessation of use, and withdrawal symptoms do not occur [85].

Effects on Children In the 1960s and 70s articles began to appear about possible teratogenic effects of lysergic acid (LSD). These were mostly case reports, and most were not able to show an association between LSD ingestion and birth defects or chromosomal abnormalities. A 1970 *Pediatrics* article reported that the existing data were inconclusive [87]. There is a dearth of recent literature on the topic. There is one case report of an accidental overdose during the first trimester of pregnancy without negative effects on the fetus [37]. However, there is evidence from animal studies that hallucinogens can cause delayed intrauterine growth, embryo deaths and fetal anomalies, so it can hardly be said with confidence that these drugs are safe during pregnancy.

Interventions Supportive care and detoxification may be needed in some cases (see [32] for a detailed description of treatment). Otherwise, there are no specific interventions separate from those used generally for substance use disorders.

Inhalants

"Inhalants include a variety of volatile substances that are inhaled to produce a high. Some examples are nitrous oxide, amyl nitrite, cleaning fluids, gasoline, spray paint, computer keyboard cleaner, other aerosol sprays, felt-tip pens, and glue" [78, p. 17]. Their abuse potential derives from their action on GABA-A receptors [73] and/or *N*-methyl-*d*-aspartate (NMDA) antagonism [11].

Inhalant use is primarily a phenomenon of adolescence, with the highest rate of use (2.7%) among 12–17-year-olds, followed by 1.5% of 18–25-year-olds [78]. These substances are easily and readily available since they are legally sold, relatively inexpensive and do not involve penalties for possession. Chronic inhalant use is associated with severe neurocognitive deficits, often irreversible. Of particular concern is the rapid development of dependence and the potential lethality of these substances even with one time use.

Inhalants tend to be most used by low income and marginalized[1] teens. While there are no data on inhalant abuse among pregnant teens, it is inevitable that some will occur in this group.

Effects on Children Given their toxicity, it is not surprising that these substances have noxious effects in utero and afterwards. A fetal solvent syndrome (FSS) has been described in association with high levels of exposure to solvents. This includes developmental problems, physical malformations such as microcephaly, prematurity, low birth weight, and fetal death [11]. After birth, infants can have growth retardation, hyperactivity, language impairments, and cerebellar dysfunction. A withdrawal syndrome has also been reported, consisting of high-pitched crying, sleeplessness, hyperactive Moro reflex, tremor and hypotonia, and difficulty in feeding [80].

Interventions Treatment for inhalant misuse has not been well studied. Acutely, detoxification and medical monitoring are the usual approaches. Positive results have been reported for family therapy, motivational interviewing, and cognitive behavioral therapy [62].

[1] "Marginalization" refers to exclusion from social, economic, and/or educational opportunities (owing to economic inequality, violence, stigma, racism, migration), family factors (including neglect and abuse), and individual factors (e.g., disability, ethnicity; [5]).

Discussion and Clinical Guidance

Recommendations for addressing substance abuse in pregnancy fall into the categories of screening, assessment, and interventions. Pregnancy offers a unique opportunity to intervene in substance use disorders. Pregnant women have a new perspective on themselves and a focus on their unborn child. This can provide a strong motivation for them to reduce or eliminate their use of substances that are potentially harmful to themselves as well as their unborn child.

Several major professional organizations have recommendations for screening, assessment, and treatment of substance use disorders in pregnant women. A joint policy statement issued by the Society for Maternal-Fetal Medicine, the American College of Obstetricians and Gynecologists, and the American Society of Addiction Medicine recommended universal screening for all women at the time of the first prenatal visit using a validated assessment instrument [27]. Canadian guidelines for pregnant adolescents also recommend "routine and repeated screening" for alcohol and drug use [31, p. 41].

Many of the instruments and interventions used have not been studied specifically in pregnant women [18] much less in pregnant adolescents, but they are the best that are available at this point. For example, the American College of Obstetrics and Gynecology recommends using the CRAFFT screening tool for pregnant adolescents. This is a tool that has been well validated for adolescents but has not been studied in pregnant adolescents. Nevertheless, this recommendation carries the weight of expert consensus, which provides the best available guidance in the absence of evidence based on clinical trials.

In 2014, the World Health Organization (WHO), citing substance abuse among pregnant and parenting women as a worldwide public health problem, issued a report based on a systematic review of published research on screening, assessment, and treatment. The report noted a low quality of evidence for all the interventions they reviewed. Nonetheless, they made several recommendations in each of these categories, based on the lack of potential harm of the intervention and the low resources required for implementation.

Identification of substance abuse is the first crucial step in intervening. The repetition of questions about substance use at each health care encounter increases the likelihood of detecting substance abuse, as patients are more likely to disclose this after they develop a trusting relationship with their health care worker and have overcome their fears of criticism and stigmatization, being reported to authorities, and losing their children if they disclose substance use [90].

But identification is only the first step. In the words of the WHO, "Appropriate intensive treatment needs to be made available for referral when substance use/alcohol use is identified and long-term, sustainable support is required" [90, p 24].

The good news is that brief interventions can be efficacious. These involve a structured, time-limited interaction. They may educate patients about the nature and dangers of substance abuse and possible warning signs of dependency. For example, a single-session brief intervention that used a 40-min manualized interview has been shown to reduce substance abuse in pregnant adolescent girls with a substance use disorder [88].

Motivational interviewing has been widely used as a key intervention for substance abuse. A key aspect of motivational interviewing is meeting patients where they are and understanding their perspective. The first step is determining readiness for change and subsequent interventions proceed from this determination. This contrasts with a paternalistic approach, which might warn of dangers and advise cessation of drug use but fail to consider the patient's own perspectives. Motivational interviewing was not recommended by the WHO owing to their conclusion that there was lack of sufficient evidence for efficacy, but the research they cited compared it with treatment as usual, which may itself have included some motivational interviewing. MI is best viewed as a first step on the pathway to treatment. Other treatment approaches include cognitive behavioral therapy, motivational enhancement therapy, contingency management, and community reinforcement. The US Substance Abuse and Mental Health Services Administration [79] found strong evidence in favor of motivational interviewing, contingency reinforcement, cognitive behavioral therapy, and community reinforcement approaches as treatments for substance abuse disorders.

Additional recommended treatment during the pregnancy includes assistance with prenatal care, cognitive behavioral therapy, parenting support, and 12-step programs.

Medication-assisted treatment, which combines pharmacological approaches with psychosocial intervention, is the standard of care for many substance use disorders. Management of withdrawal symptoms may also be necessary. Psychopharmacological medications may be needed for psychiatric symptoms.

Salas-Wight and Wu in the review cited above [72] found consistent parental support and academic engagement were protective against substance use among pregnant teens. This suggests that providing support to parents of teen mothers and implementing school programs to support academic engagement would be important interventions. Parenting support is also likely to be necessary. We will discuss interventions to support pregnant and parenting teens in a later chapter.

As new mothers with a history of substance abuse face risks of losing their children if they relapse, there are important incentives for them to adhere to mandated treatment, including regular drug testing. At the same time, concerns about criminal prosecution and loss of custody of their children deter women from disclosing substance abuse and seeking help. As urged by the American College of Obstetrics and Gynecology, "Seeking obstetric–gynecologic care should not expose a woman to criminal or civil penalties for marijuana use, such as incarceration, involuntary commitment, loss of custody of her children, or loss of housing" [19].

Continued treatment of substance abuse after pregnancy is crucial. As noted in the World Health Organization report:

> Alcohol use, binge drinking, tobacco and cannabis use rates rebound substantially in the postpartum period compared with use during pregnancy. Depression correlates with substance use, and new mothers with postpartum depression may be at high risk for substance

use or return to substance use. Maternal psychopathology is more common in substance-dependent women than in the general population, and is not infrequently related to poor judgment, enhancing the physical risk to the infant. [90, p. 15].

Conclusion

In summary, substance abuse not only has adverse effects on the developing fetus, many of which persist long after birth, it also interferes with parenting in a way that is highly detrimental to children and frequently results in out of home placement.

There are many shared risk factors for substance abuse and unintended pregnancy. Nonetheless, while substance use may place adolescents at risk for early or unintended pregnancy, the fact that many are able to stop their use during pregnancy out of concern for the health of their unborn child points to pregnancy as a critical period for intervention. Interventions should be partnerships in which the young mother-to-be is an active participant. Understanding the perspective of the pregnant adolescent and new mother is crucial for tailoring efficacious interventions. In the words of one researcher, "We need to do a better job of knowing patients' perspectives before we try to get them to adopt healthier behaviors" [6].

References

1. Abel EL. An update on incidence of FAS: FAS is not an equal opportunity birth defect. Neurotoxicol Teratol. 1995;17(4):437–43. https://doi.org/10.1016/0892-0362(95)00005-c.
2. Ahmadi-Montecalvo H, Haile ZT, Umer A, Chertok IRA. Adolescent pregnancy and smoking in West Virginia: pregnancy risk assessment monitoring system (PRAMS) 2005–2010. Matern Child Health J. 2016;20(12):2465–73. https://doi.org/10.1007/s10995-016-2040-y.
3. American Psychiatric Association. Diagnostic and statistical manual of mental disorders: DSM-5TM, 5th ed. (2013-14907-000). American Psychiatric Publishing Inc; 2013. https://doi.org/10.1176/appi.books.9780890425596.
4. Asante KO, Nelms-Matzke J. Survey of children with chronic handicaps and fetal alcohol syndrome in the Yukon and Northwest BC. Ottawa: Department of Welfare; 1985.
5. Auerswald CL, Piatt AA, Mirzazadeh A. Research with disadvantaged, vulnerable and/or marginalized adolescents. In: Innocenti Research Briefs 2017- 06, Methods: Conducting Research with Adolescents in Low- and Middle-Income Countries, no. 4. Innocenti: UNICEF Office of Research; 2017.
6. Barbosa-Leiker C, Burduli E, Smith C, Brooks O, Orr M, Gartstein M. Daily cannabis use during pregnancy and postpartum in a state with legalized recreational cannabis. J Addict Med. 2020;14:101306759. https://doi.org/10.1097/ADM.0000000000000625.
7. Benowitz NL. Nicotine addiction. N Engl J Med. 2010;362(24):2295–303. https://doi.org/10.1056/NEJMra0809890.
8. Bingol N, Schuster C, Fuchs M, Iosub S, Turner G, Stone RK, Gromisch DS. The influence of socioeconomic factors on the occurrence of fetal alcohol syndrome. Adv Alcohol Subst Abuse. 1987;6(4):105–18. https://doi.org/10.1300/J251v06n04_08.
9. Black AY, Fleming NA, Rome ES. Pregnancy in adolescents. Adolesc Med State Art Rev. 2012;23(1):38, xi.
10. Bottorff JL, Poole N, Kelly MT, Greaves L, Marcellus L, Jung M. Tobacco and alcohol use in the context of adolescent pregnancy and postpartum: a scoping review of the literature. Health Soc Care Community. 2014;22(6):561–74. https://doi.org/10.1111/hsc.12091.

11. Bowen SE. Two serious and challenging medical complications associated with volatile substance misuse: sudden sniffing death and fetal solvent syndrome. Subst Use Misuse. 2011;46(Suppl 1):68–72. https://doi.org/10.3109/10826084.2011.580220.
12. Carey KB, Guthrie KM, Rich CM, Krieger NH, Norris AL, Kaplan C, Carey MP. Alcohol use and sexual risk behavior in young women: a qualitative study. AIDS Behav. 2019;23(6):1647–55. https://doi.org/10.1007/s10461-018-2310-3.
13. Centers for Disease Control and Prevention. Annual surveillance report of drug-related risks and outcomes—United States, Surveillance Special Report. Atanta: Centers for Disease Control and Prevention; 2018.
14. Chamberlain C, O'Mara-Eves A, Porter J, Coleman T, Perlen SM, Thomas J, McKenzie JE. Psychosocial interventions for supporting women to stop smoking in pregnancy. Cochrane Database Syst Rev. 2017;2(2):CD001055. https://doi.org/10.1002/14651858.CD001055.pub5.
15. Chan B, Freeman M, Kondo K, Ayers C, Montgomery J, Paynter R, Kansagara D. Pharmacotherapy for methamphetamine/amphetamine use disorder-a systematic review and meta-analysis. Addiction. 2019;114(12):2122–36. https://doi.org/10.1111/add.14755.
16. Charlotte W, Loshak H, Dulong C. Withdrawal management and treatment of crystal methamphetamine addiction in pregnancy: a review of clinical effectiveness and guidelines. Ottawa: Canadian Agency for Drugs and Technologies in Health; 2019. Retrieved from: https://www.ncbi.nlm.nih.gov/books/NBK546255/
17. Claire R, Chamberlain C, Davey M-A, Cooper SE, Berlin I, Leonardi-Bee J, Coleman T. Pharmacological interventions for promoting smoking cessation during pregnancy. Cochrane Database Syst Rev. 2020;3(3):CD010078. https://doi.org/10.1002/14651858.CD010078.pub3.
18. Coleman-Cowger VH, Oga EA, Peters EN, Trocin KE, Koszowski B, Mark K. Accuracy of three screening tools for prenatal substance use. Obstet Gynecol. 2019;133(5):952–61. https://doi.org/10.1097/AOG.0000000000003230.
19. Committee Opinion No. 633: Alcohol abuse and other substance use disorders: ethical issues in obstetric and gynecologic practice. Obstet Gynecol. 2015;125(6):1529–37. https://doi.org/10.1097/01.AOG.0000466371.86393.9b
20. Committee Opinion No. 722: Marijuana use during pregnancy and lactation. Obstet Gynecol. 2017;130(4):e205–9. https://doi.org/10.1097/AOG.0000000000002354
21. Constantine NA, Slater JK, Carroll JA, Antin TMJ. Smoking cessation, maintenance, and relapse experiences among pregnant and postpartum adolescents: a qualitative analysis. J Adolesc Health. 2014;55(2):216–21. https://doi.org/10.1016/j.jadohealth.2013.12.027.
22. Cornelius MD, Day NL. Developmental consequences of prenatal tobacco exposure. Curr Opin Neurol. 2009;22(2):121–5. https://doi.org/10.1097/WCO.0b013e328326f6dc.
23. Cornelius MD, Goldschmidt L, DeGenna N, Day NL. Smoking during teenage pregnancies: Effects on behavioral problems in offspring. Nicotine Tob Res. 2007;9(7):739–50. https://doi.org/10.1080/14622200701416971.
24. Dodge P, Nadolski K, Kopkau H, Zablocki V, Forrestal K, Bailey BA. The impact of timing of in utero marijuana exposure on fetal growth. Front Pediatr. 2023;11:1103749. https://doi.org/10.3389/fped.2023.1103749. PMID: 37260795; PMCID: PMC10228645.
25. Doherty E, Wiggers J, Wolfenden L, Anderson AE, Crooks K, Tsang TW, Kingsland M. Antenatal care for alcohol consumption during pregnancy: pregnant women's reported receipt of care and associated characteristics. BMC Pregnancy Childbirth. 2019;19(1):299. https://doi.org/10.1186/s12884-019-2436-y.
26. Dyba J, Moesgen D, Klein M, Leyendecker B. Methamphetamine use in German Families: parental substance use, parent-child interaction and risks for children involved. Subst Use Misuse. 2019;54(4):583–91. https://doi.org/10.1080/10826084.2018.1528459.
27. Ecker J, Abuhamad A, Hill W, Bailit J, Bateman BT, Berghella V, Yonkers KA. Substance use disorders in pregnancy: clinical, ethical, and research imperatives of the opioid epidemic: a report of a joint workshop of the Society for Maternal-Fetal Medicine, American College of Obstetricians and Gynecologists, and American Society of Addiction Medicine. Am J Obstet Gynecol. 2019;221(1):B5–B28. https://doi.org/10.1016/j.ajog.2019.03.022.

28. Elliott TE, Frail CK, Pawloski PA, Thomas AJ, Werner AM, Rossom RC. Opioid use during pregnancy, observations of opioid use, and secular trend from 2006 to 2014 at HealthPartners Medical Group. Clin J Pain. 2018;34(8):707–12.
29. Embry D, Hankins M, Biglan A, Boles S. Behavioral and social correlates of methamphetamine use in a population-based sample of early and later adolescents. Addict Behav. 2009;34(4):343–51. https://doi.org/10.1016/j.addbeh.2008.11.019.
30. Fanshawe TR, Halliwell W, Lindson N, Aveyard P, Livingstone-Banks J, Hartmann-Boyce J. Tobacco cessation interventions for young people. Cochrane Database Syst Rev. 2017;11(11):CD003289. https://doi.org/10.1002/14651858.CD003289.pub6.
31. Fleming N, O'Driscoll T, Becker G, Spitzer RF. Adolescent pregnancy guidelines. J Obstet Gynaecol Can. 2015;37(8):740–56. https://doi.org/10.1016/S1701-2163(15)30180-8.
32. Forest JS. Hallucinogen use. Medscape; 2020. https://emedicine.medscape.com/article/293752-overview
33. Gentzke AS, Creamer M, Cullen KA, Ambrose BK, Willis G, Jamal A, King BA. Vital signs: tobacco product use among middle and high school students—United States, 2011-2018. MMWR Morb Mortal Wkly Rep. 2019;68(6):157–64. https://doi.org/10.15585/mmwr.mm6806e1.
34. Gentzke AS, Wang TW, Jamal A, Park-Lee E, Ren C, Cullen KA, Neff L. Tobacco product use among middle and high school students—United States, 2020. MMWR Morb Mortal Wkly Rep. 2020;69(50):1881–8. https://doi.org/10.15585/mmwr.mm6950a1.
35. Gray KM. New developments in understanding and treating adolescent marijuana dependence. Adolesc Psychiatry. 2013;3(4):297–306. https://doi.org/10.2174/221067660304140121173215.
36. Gunn JKL, Rosales CB, Center KE, Nuñez A, Gibson SJ, Christ C, Ehiri JE. Prenatal exposure to cannabis and maternal and child health outcomes: a systematic review and meta-analysis. BMJ Open. 2016;6(4):e009986. https://doi.org/10.1136/bmjopen-2015-009986.
37. Haden M, Woods B. LSD overdoses: three case reports. J Stud Alcohol Drugs. 2020;81(1):115–8.
38. Hamel C, Corace K, Hersi M, Rice D, Willows M, Macpherson P, Sproule B, Flores-Aranda J, Garber G, Esmaeilisaraji L, Skidmore B, Porath A, Ortiz Nunez R, Hutton B. Psychosocial and pharmacologic interventions for methamphetamine addiction: protocol for a scoping review of the literature. Syst Rev. 2020;9(1):245. https://doi.org/10.1186/s13643-020-01499-z.
39. Harlow AF, Wesselink AK, Hatch EE, Rothman KJ, Wise LA. Male preconception marijuana use and spontaneous abortion: a prospective cohort study. Epidemiology. 2021;32(2):239–47. https://doi.org/10.1097/EDE.0000000000001303. PMID: 33165011; PMCID: PMC7855868.
40. Hayer S, Mandelbaum AD, Watch L, Ryan KS, Hedges MA, Manuzak JA, Easley CA 4th, Schust DJ, Lo JO. Cannabis and pregnancy: a review. Obstet Gynecol Surv. 2023;78(7):411–28. https://doi.org/10.1097/OGX.0000000000001159. PMID: 37480292; PMCID: PMC10372687.
41. Hensley L, Sulo S, Kozmic S, Parilla B. Opioid addiction in pregnancy: Does depression negatively impact adherence with prenatal care? J Addict Med. 2018;12:101306759. https://doi.org/10.1097/ADM.0000000000000364.
42. Huizink AC, Mulder EJH. Maternal smoking, drinking or cannabis use during pregnancy and neurobehavioral and cognitive functioning in human offspring. Neurosci Biobehav Rev. 2006;30(1):24–41. https://doi.org/10.1016/j.neubiorev.2005.04.005.
43. Jones KL, Smith DW. Recognition of the fetal alcohol syndrome in early infancy. Lancet. 1973;302(7836):999–1001. https://doi.org/10.1016/s0140-6736(73)91092-1.
44. Jones HE, Kaltenbach K, Heil SH, Stine SM, Coyle MG, Arria AM, O'Grady KE, Selby P, Martin PR, Fischer G. Neonatal abstinence syndrome after methadone or buprenorphine exposure. N Engl J Med. 2010;363(24):2320–31. https://doi.org/10.1056/NEJMoa1005359.
45. Kalaitzopoulos DR, Chatzistergiou K, Amylidi AL, Kokkinidis D, Goulis D, MD, P. Effect of methamphetamine hydrochloride on pregnancy outcome: a systematic review and meta-analysis. J Addict Med. 2018;12(3):220–6. https://doi.org/10.1097/ADM.0000000000000391.
46. Kazemi T, Huang S, Avci NG, Waits CMK, Akay YM, Akay M. Investigating the influence of perinatal nicotine and alcohol exposure on the genetic profiles of dopaminergic neurons in the VTA using miRNA-mRNA analysis. Sci Rep. 2020;10(1):15016. https://doi.org/10.1038/s41598-020-71875-1.

47. Kharbanda EO, Vazquez-Benitez G, Kunin-Batson A, Nordin JD, Olsen A, Romitti PA. Birth and early developmental screening outcomes associated with cannabis exposure during pregnancy. J Perinatol. 2020;40(3):473–80. https://doi.org/10.1038/s41372-019-0576-6.
48. Ko JY, Farr SL, Tong VT, Creanga AA, Callaghan WM. Prevalence and patterns of marijuana use among pregnant and nonpregnant women of reproductive age. Am J Obstet Gynecol. 2015;213(2):201.e1–10. https://doi.org/10.1016/j.ajog.2015.03.021.
49. Kondo KK, Morasco BJ, Nugent SM, Ayers CK, O'Neil ME, Freeman M, Kansagara D. Pharmacotherapy for the treatment of cannabis use disorder: a systematic review. Ann Intern Med. 2020;172(6):398–412. https://doi.org/10.7326/M19-1105.
50. Kotchick BA, Shaffer A, Forehand R, Miller KS. Adolescent sexual risk behavior: a multi-system perspective. Clin Psychol Rev. 2001;21(4):493–519. https://doi.org/10.1016/s0272-7358(99)00070-7.
51. Larcombe AN. Early-life exposure to electronic cigarettes: cause for concern. Lancet Respir Med. 2019;7(11):985–92. https://doi.org/10.1016/S2213-2600(19)30189-4.
52. Lowe CR. Effect of mothers' smoking habits on birth weight of their children. Br Med J. 1959;2(5153):673–6. https://doi.org/10.1136/bmj.2.5153.673.
53. May PA, Gossage JP. Maternal risk factors for fetal alcohol spectrum disorders: not as simple as it might seem. Alcohol Res Health. 2011;34(1):15–26.
54. McGuinness TM, Pollack D. Parental methamphetamine abuse and children. J Pediatr Health Care. 2008;22(3):152–8. https://doi.org/10.1016/j.pedhc.2007.04.009.
55. McQuire C, Daniel R, Hurt L, Kemp A, Paranjothy S. The causal web of foetal alcohol spectrum disorders: a review and causal diagram. Eur Child Adolesc Psychiatry. 2020;29(5):575–94. https://doi.org/10.1007/s00787-018-1264-3.
56. Meyer M, Johnston A, Crocker A, Heil S. Methadone and Buprenorphine for Opioid dependence during pregnancy: a retrospective cohort study. J Addict Med. 2015;9(2):81–6. https://doi.org/10.1097/ADM.0000000000000092.
57. Miech RA, Schulenberg JE, Johnston LD, Bachman JG, O'Malley PM, Patrick ME. National adolescent drug trends in 2019: findings released. Ann Arbor: Institute for Social Research, The University of Michigan; 2019.
58. Nagpal TS, Green CR, Cook JL. Vaping during pregnancy: what are the potential health outcomes and perceptions pregnant women have? J Obstet Gynaecol Canada. 2020; https://doi.org/10.1016/j.jogc.2020.05.014.
59. Natale BV, Gustin KN, Lee K, Holloway AC, Laviolette SR, Natale DRC, Hardy DB. Δ9-tetrahydrocannabinol exposure during rat pregnancy leads to symmetrical fetal growth restriction and labyrinth-specific vascular defects in the placenta. Sci Rep. 2020;10(1):544. https://doi.org/10.1038/s41598-019-57318-6.
60. National Center for Chronic Disease Prevention and Health Promotion (US) Office on Smoking and Health. Preventing tobacco use among youth and young adults: a report of the surgeon general. Atlanta (GA): Centers for Disease Control and Prevention (US); 2012. https://www.ncbi.nlm.nih.gov/books/NBK99237/.
61. National Institute on Alcohol Abuse and Alcoholism. What is binge drinking? Rockville: Author; 2020. Retrieved from https://www.niaaa.nih.gov/publications/brochures-and-fact-sheets/binge-drinking
62. Nguyen J, O'Brien C, Schapp S. Adolescent inhalant use prevention, assessment, and treatment: a literature synthesis. Int J Drug Policy. 2016;31:15–24. https://doi.org/10.1016/j.drugpo.2016.02.001.
63. Nichols DE, Grob CS. Is LSD toxic? Forensic Sci Int. 2018;284:141–5. https://doi.org/10.1016/j.forsciint.2018.01.006.
64. Paul SE, Hatoum AS, Fine JD, Johnson EC, Hansen I, Karcher NR, Moreau AL, Bondy E, Qu Y, Carter EB, Rogers CE, Agrawal A, Barch DM, Bogdan R. Associations between prenatal cannabis exposure and childhood outcomes: results from the ABCD study. JAMA Psychiatry. 2021;78(1):64–76. https://doi.org/10.1001/jamapsychiatry.2020.2902. PMID: 32965490; PMCID: PMC7512132.

65. Perez-Reyes M, Wall ME. Presence of delta9-tetrahydrocannabinol in human milk. N Engl J Med. 1982;307(13):819–20. https://doi.org/10.1056/NEJM198209233071311.
66. Pesko MF, Currie JM. E-cigarette minimum legal sale age laws and traditional cigarette use among rural pregnant teenagers. J Health Econ. 2019;66:71–90. https://doi.org/10.1016/j.jhealeco.2019.05.003.
67. Popova S, Lange S, Probst C, Gmel G, Rehm J. Estimation of national, regional, and global prevalence of alcohol use during pregnancy and fetal alcohol syndrome: a systematic review and meta-analysis. Lancet Glob Health. 2017;5(3):e290–9. https://doi.org/10.1016/S2214-109X(17)30021-9.
68. Poulin C, Graham L. The association between substance use, unplanned sexual intercourse and other sexual behaviours among adolescent students. Addiction. 2001;96(4):607–21. https://doi.org/10.1046/j.1360-0443.2001.9646079.x.
69. Prince MK, Ayers D. Substance use in pregnancy. *StatPearls*. Treasure Island: StatPearls Publishing; 2020. Retrieved from: https://www.ncbi.nlm.nih.gov/books/NBK542330
70. Roddy E. Bupropion and other non-nicotine pharmacotherapies. BMJ (Clinical Research Ed). 2004;328(7438):509–11. https://doi.org/10.1136/bmj.328.7438.509.
71. Roncero C, Valriberas-Herrero I, Mezzatesta-Gava M, Villegas JL, Aguilar L, Grau-López L. Cannabis use during pregnancy and its relationship with fetal developmental outcomes and psychiatric disorders. A systematic review. Reprod Health. 2020;17(1):25. https://doi.org/10.1186/s12978-020-0880-9.
72. Salas-Wright CP, Vaughn MG, Ugalde J, Todic J. Substance use and teen pregnancy in the United States: evidence from the NSDUH. Addict Behav. 2015;45:218–25. https://doi.org/10.1016/j.addbeh.2015.01.039.
73. Shelton KL. Discriminative stimulus effects of abused inhalants. Curr Top Behav Neurosci. 2018;39:113–39.
74. Simpson WJ. A preliminary report on cigarette smoking and the incidence of prematurity. Am J Obstet Gynecol. 1957;73(4):807–15.
75. Sithisarn T, Granger DT, Bada HS. Consequences of prenatal substance use. Int J Adolesc Med Health. 2012;24(2):105–12. https://doi.org/10.1515/ijamh.2012.016.
76. Smid MC, Metz TD, Gordon AJ. Stimulant use in pregnancy: an under-recognized epidemic among pregnant women. Clin Obstet Gynecol. 2019;62(1):168–84. https://doi.org/10.1097/GRF.0000000000000418.
77. Sood B, Delaney-Black V, Covington C, Nordstrom-Klee B, Ager J, Templin T, Janisse J, Martier S, Sokol RJ. Prenatal alcohol exposure and childhood behavior at age 6 to 7 years: I. dose-response effect. Pediatrics. 2001;108(2):E34. https://doi.org/10.1542/peds.108.2.e34.
78. Substance Abuse and Mental Health Services Administration. Key substance use and mental health indicators in the United States: results from the 2018 National Survey on Drug Use and Health, HHS Publication No. PEP19-5068, NSDUH Series H-54. Rockville: Center for Behavioral Health Statistics and Quality, Substance Abuse and Mental Health Services Administration; 2019. https://www.samhsa.gov/data/
79. Substance Abuse and Mental Health Services Administration. Treatment of stimulant use disorders, SAMHSA Publication No. PEP20-06-01-001. Rockville: National Mental Health and Substance Use Policy Laboratory; 2020.
80. Tenenbein M, Casiro OG, Seshia MM, Debooy VD. Neonatal withdrawal from maternal volatile substance abuse. Arch Dis Child Fetal Neonat Educ. 1996;74(3):F204–7.
81. Tobon AL, Habecker E, Forray A. Opioid use in pregnancy. Curr Psychiatry Rep. 2019;21(12):118. https://doi.org/10.1007/s11920-019-1110-4.
82. Towers CV, Katz E, Weitz B, Visconti K. Use of naltrexone in treating opioid use disorder in pregnancy. Am J Obstet Gynecol. 2020;222(1):83.e1–8. https://doi.org/10.1016/j.ajog.2019.07.037.
83. Tran DT, Preen DB, Einarsdottir K, Kemp-Casey A, Randall D, Jorm LR, Choi SKY, Havard A. Use of smoking cessation pharmacotherapies during pregnancy is not associated with

increased risk of adverse pregnancy outcomes: a population-based cohort study. BMC Med. 2020;18(1):15. https://doi.org/10.1186/s12916-019-1472-9.
84. Turner E, Jones M, Vaz LR, Coleman T. Systematic review and meta-analysis to assess the safety of bupropion and varenicline in pregnancy. Nicotine Tob Res. 2019;21(8):1001–10. https://doi.org/10.1093/ntr/nty055.
85. US Dept of Health and Human Services, National Institutes of Health. Hallucinogens and dissociative drugs NIDA Research Report Series, NIH Publication Number 15-4209 • Revised February 2015. https://www.drugabuse.gov/sites/default/files/rrhalluc.pdf
86. Volkow ND, Han B, Compton WM, Blanco C. Marijuana use during stages of pregnancy in the United States. Ann Intern Med. 2017;166(10):763–4. https://doi.org/10.7326/L17-0067.
87. Warren RJ, Rimoin DL, Sly WS. LSD exposure in utero. Pediatrics. 1970;45(3):466–9.
88. Whicher E, Utku F, Schirmer G, Davis P, Abou-Saleh M. Pilot project to evaluate the effectiveness and acceptability of single-session brief counseling for the prevention of substance misuse in pregnant adolescents. Addict Disord Treat. 2012;11:43–9. https://doi.org/10.1097/ADT.0b013e3182387029.
89. Wolfson L, Schmidt RA, Stinson J, Poole N. Examining barriers to harm reduction and child welfare services for pregnant women and mothers who use substances using a stigma action framework. Health Soc Care Community. 2021; https://doi.org/10.1111/hsc.13335.
90. World Health Organization. Guidelines for the identification and management of substance use and substance use disorders in pregnancy. Geneva: Author; 2014. Retrieved from https://www.who.int/publications/i/item/9789241548731
91. Wright TE, Schuetter R, Tellei J, Sauvage L. Methamphetamines and pregnancy outcomes. J Addict Med. 2015;9(2):111–7. https://doi.org/10.1097/ADM.0000000000000101.
92. Zapata LB, Hillis SD, Marchbanks PA, Curtis KM, Lowry R. Methamphetamine use is independently associated with recent risky sexual behaviors and adolescent pregnancy. J Sch Health. 2008;78(12):641–8. https://doi.org/10.1111/j.1746-1561.2008.00360.x.

Implications for Public Policy Toward Teen Pregnancy and Parenting

10

Gordon Harper and Lois T. Flaherty

Introduction

Public policy is an institutionalized way of solving problems perceived as pressing and in need of organized solutions. It involves conceptualizing the problem and developing and implementing a solution. Policies can be developed and implemented in a top-down manner, by government decree, or can be formulated with input from various stakeholders. Historically policies affecting vulnerable populations have not been developed in collaboration with members of these groups. Public policy regarding teen pregnancy has reflected deeply felt attitudes toward teen sexual activity and toward those teens who may become pregnant or parents. These attitudes, though not always overtly acknowledged, shape how policy is developed. They can reinforce social stigma, hurting the intended beneficiaries. They can also restrict access to resources [cf. 8].

On the other hand, policy can support and empower young parents in their roles as parents and as emerging adults. The implementation of policies related to teen pregnancy and parenting can provide important resources, especially to vulnerable populations of young parents and their children. This requires a change in the paradigm by which we understand the phenomenon of teen pregnancy and parenting. This chapter will review both aspects of public policy and discuss how emerging paradigms are changing it.

Public policy arises out of perceptions of problems, their root causes, and their solutions. Ideally these perceptions should be based on the best available evidence, but this is certainly often far from the case. We saw in chapter one how perceptions of an epidemic of teen pregnancy in the 1990s were associated with beliefs, without evidence, that teenagers were deliberately having babies in order to get financial support from welfare programs. The perceived solution was to cut back on welfare

G. Harper · L. T. Flaherty (✉)
Harvard Medical School and Cambridge Health Alliance, Cambridge, MA, USA
e-mail: gordon_harper@hms.harvard.edu

J.-V. P. Wittenberg et al. (eds.), *Adolescent Pregnancy and Parenting*,
https://doi.org/10.1007/978-3-031-42502-8_10

benefits. The result was an increase in child poverty rather than a decrease in out of wedlock birth.

Negative perceptions of young mothers go beyond the idea that they are free-loaders, however. The "evidence" supporting these views was generated by decades of flawed research on outcomes of teen pregnancy, which we have discussed in other chapters in this book.

This research showing negative outcomes has supported a negative and pessimistic view that teen parents are doomed to poverty, low educational achievement, and dependency on public welfare, and that their children are doomed to replicate these outcomes. This has reinforced a pejorative view of teens who allow themselves to become pregnant and give birth. The prevailing view has been the only way to avoid these dismal outcomes is to prevent teen pregnancy. While it is desirable to prevent unwanted pregnancies in general, the emphasis in public policy has been mainly on prevention through education, increased access to contraception, and abstinence, with relatively little attention being given to ameliorating the social circumstances that place adolescents at risk.

However, as we have pointed out, much of this research was guided by negative cultural attitudes, which then found support in the "evidence" on outcomes of teen pregnancy. Much of the research failed to account for the context of pre-existing psychosocial adversity that both increases the likelihood of teen pregnancy and contributes to negative outcomes. Furthermore, outcomes are not universally negative, as we saw in the chapter on lived experience, where we heard the stories of young mothers who succeeded in raising their children at the same time that they worked to become independent adults. Nonetheless it is the unitary, negative view of young pregnancy and parenthood that has often guided public policy. Such a view fails to account for the full range of outcomes and ignores the circumstances in which pregnancy and parenthood can have positive effects on the young and the highly variable cultural context in which pregnancy and parenthood occur, as well as the circumstances in which pregnancy and parenthood can have positive effects on the young – and in which more differentiated knowledge of outcomes is needed.

Cultural Attitudes and Paradigms

Attitudes that are shared, but not necessarily widely acknowledged, are examples of what Kuhn called "dominant paradigms" (1970). He argued that such paradigms, mostly unrecognized, shape the way social phenomena get perceived, discussed, and studied**.** They embody hidden assumptions. In science, researchers' preconceptions affect how phenomena are studied, the types of experiments that are done, the collection of data, and the conclusions that are drawn from the results. Paradigm shifts occur when new evidence emerges that challenges the validity of the existing views. One example is the Ptolemaic view that the Sun revolves around the stationary "center of the universe" – the Earth, a theory that fell as a consequence of Copernicus' observations.

Regarding teen pregnancy and parenting, the dominant paradigm has seen it as a unitary phenomenon, in conflict with cultural mores and therefore shameful, as well as adversely affecting the health development of mothers and children. These generally held views have dominated research and public policy in the USA. They have been accepted as certainties without attention being paid to conflicting evidence based on the voices of those actually affected – those with lived experience (both the parents and their children). They have reinforced the social stigma of teen pregnancy. They have failed to consider ways to address the *actual* needs of those affected. Most importantly, they have resulted in "evidence" that supports negative and stigmatizing views of teen parents.

As has happened with other stigmatized conditions, like HIV/AIDS, when the factual basis of stigmatizing beliefs is contradicted by new data, the existing paradigm can be challenged, and a *paradigm shift* occurs [10]. But when such a paradigm, in society in general and among professionals, is not acknowledged, let alone challenged, social stigma is reinforced.

"Perverse Incentives"

One of the paradigms influencing policies for supporting families and children is the belief in perverse incentives. A perverse incentive is a policy that has unintended consequences that are the opposite of the goal of the policy. An often-cited example is the so-called cobra effect, in which people in India started breeding cobras after a bounty was offered for their capture, and then released them into the wild after the bounty ended [15]. One of the arguments made for policies that offer little help and considerable shame to young parents is that support will act as a perverse incentive to increase the frequency of the cited behavior – in other words, supporting young parents will encourage teen pregnancy and parenthood. In the USA, this argument underlay the termination, in the 1990s, of the program called Aid to Families with Dependent Children (AFDC). This program had for 60 years provided financial support for needy parents of young children. In the debates leading to the termination of such supports, phrases like "encouraging dependency" and "irresponsible behavior" were often heard. Over the years, the policy goal shifted from helping poor mothers stay at home with their young children to getting such women into the workforce, policy promoted as decreasing the "welfare rolls." The well-being, current or future, of children or parents, did not figure in these debates. As a result, in 1994 AFDC was replaced by TANF (Transitional Assistance to Needy Families). While some fiscal conservatives were satisfied with this change, debate continues as to the effects on children and families, notably, the increase of children growing up in poverty [6].

The paradigm of perverse incentives has strong racial undertones. Dyck and Hussey [5], writing about the influence of racial attitudes on welfare policy, point out that despite evidence that the fact that "the nature of the information environment surrounding welfare policy has fundamentally changed," stereotypes about welfare recipients being lazy and disinclined to work have persisted. They examined media coverage of poor people and found a trend toward less racial stereotyping, and more accurate depictions of the poor population as being diverse. This was not, however, reflected in corresponding shifts in racial attitudes on the part of the public as measured by surveys. This suggests that more than evidence is needed to drive public policy.

Non-acknowledgment Is Ineffective Policy

What if we examine cultural attitudes and political ideology in terms of measurable outcomes achieved? What is known about the effects of policy? Simply put, policies based on shame and stigma do *not* reduce pregnancy rates – quite the opposite. Not acknowledging something may reflect a magical belief in the power of avoidance: what is not discussed will not happen. This lack of acknowledgment lies behind opposition to both sex education and access to contraception – the belief, despite evidence to the contrary, is that teaching children and adolescents about sex and how to avoid pregnancy will encourage them to have sex. Sex education laws and policies are developed at the state and local level. Although 32 states require sex education, only 22 require that it be medically accurate. Some districts advocate "abstinence only" sex education; others prohibit mention of terms such as intercourse, masturbation and abortion, and still others are required to teach that abortion is wrong [12]. In contrast, comprehensive sex education, while emphasizing that abstinence is the only sure way of avoiding pregnancy, also includes information on contraception, sexuality, and avoidance of sexually transmitted diseases.

The result of lack of access to medically accurate information is disbelief among many American teens regarding the possibility of pregnancy, and a lack of information about or access to birth control; higher rates of teen pregnancy and young births are seen in States where young people are *not* given information about sexual activity and contraception, compared to communities in which schools provide such information. This finding has been reported in both in the general literature [17] and in sociological studies [13]. A caveat to interpreting these findings is that socially conservative states have populations with less access to birth control, lower rates of high school graduation and increased religiosity, all of which are also associated with high teen birth rates, making it difficult to disentangle the effects of policy from the influence of social factors [19].

International comparisons show the same correlation. While sexual *activity* among teens is as frequent in Western Europe as it is in the USA, the rate of *pregnancy,* mostly unplanned, is 3 to 15 times higher in the USA. Countries in Western Europe generally are more open in acknowledging that sexual behavior among teens occurs, and more proactive in providing access to reproductive health care. Ignorance may feel like bliss, but it does not result in abstinence.

Need for More Than Sex Education and Prevention

Suggesting that the variability in teen pregnancy rates is due to more than unevenness in educational curricula, a Cochrane review argued for interventions going beyond education and involving affected youth in program design [11]. This review found that incentives to keep students in school had a more important impact than sex education. It advocated for supplementing what happens in school with community-based interventions, augmenting *assets* – or protective factors in the community, family, and the individual. These assets have been demonstrated to have more effect on pregnancy rates than education alone [3, 4].

For decades, American policy has focused exclusively on preventing teen pregnancy, and by implication seeing any pregnancy among young people as an adverse outcome. This exclusive emphasis has stigmatized youth who are pregnant or become parents, with negative effects on young parents and their children summarized in other chapters. That emphasis is now changing.

New Policies to Support Young People, Parents or Not

From Shame and Exclusion to Inclusion and Empowerment

New policy models are emerging. Initiatives across the country are seeing young people, not as future delinquents needing to be controlled, but as young adults with resources to be supported and risks to be addressed. These initiatives see education, including education about sexuality, as a part of empowerment.

These initiatives include young people, both those who might become pregnant and those already parents, in program development. They want to change the message within sexual education curriculums, from the old message that focuses on negative aspects of teen pregnancy and the babies born to teen parents, to one that promotes the development of young people through education, respect, and empowerment. Many of these initiatives address the entire youth population, rather than focusing exclusively on those at high risk of unplanned pregnancy. Interventions specially tailored to each group have a place but targeting only those at high risk may reinforce stigma. When intervention, including education, is directed to the entire population, no one is singled out and stigmatized. This approach resembles educational initiatives that aim to make the classroom respective and protective of all students, not only those identified as survivors of bullying, trauma or adverse childhood experiences. These initiatives are also using gender-inclusive language to make sure that young parents of all genders are receiving adequate, respectful information.

The Patient-Centered Care Movement

The Institute of Medicine defines patient-centered care as "providing care that is respectful of, and responsive to, individual patient preferences, needs and values, and ensuring that patient values guide all clinical decisions" [9, p. 6]. This approach differs from a traditional model in which the patient is a passive recipient of services. Rather, it involves a collaborative approach requiring a true partnership between individuals and their healthcare providers. Key aspects of patient-centered care are listening to what the patient says she wants and needs, providing complete information, and engaging in joint decision-making about treatment. Patients are treated as capable of autonomous and informed decisions about their care. Their cultural traditions and values are appreciated and respected. Involvement of families is encouraged. Monitoring outcomes is also an important component. Implementing this approach requires rethinking on the part of providers as well as reconfiguring health care systems.

Originally aimed at improving care for chronic conditions, patient-centered care has been shown to improve outcomes in a variety of settings and populations.

Specialty Clinics for Pregnant Adolescents

At this point there are only a handful of clinics specially designed for pregnant adolescents in the USA. Most are at major academic centers. They involve a variety of services including group sessions, classes on childbirth, parenting, and life skills, and assistance with accessing educational and vocational resources. However, several organizations have published guidelines for the care for pregnant adolescents that can be implemented in medical practices. The most comprehensive are those of the Canadian Paediatric and Adolescent Gynaecology and Obstetricians (CANPAGO) committee of the Society of Obstetricians and Gynaecologists of Canada [7]. They have a list of 23 recommendations, most of which deal with the medical management of pregnancy and its complications, but the first two, listed below, emphasize the importance of specially tailored programs for adolescents.

1. Health care providers should adapt their prenatal care for adolescents and offer multidisciplinary care that is easily accessible to the adolescent early in the pregnancy, recognizing that adolescents often present to care later than their adult counterparts. A model that provides an opportunity to address all of these needs at one site may be the preferred model of care for pregnant adolescents (II-1A).
2. Health care providers should be sensitive to the unique developmental needs of adolescents through all stages of pregnancy and during intrapartum and postpartum care. (III-B).

Focus on Preventing *Unintended* Pregnancy

Representative of these new initiatives is a new movement, shifting from preventing *any* teen pregnancies to preventing *unplanned* teen pregnancies. The National Campaign to Prevent Unintended Pregnancy, a national organization that develops federal policies to prevent teenage pregnancy, was renamed Power to Decide. The name change is consistent with efforts to *empower* young people, giving them information and means to make their own choices.

Given the frequency of repeat pregnancies among teens, counseling about contraception post-delivery is a universally agreed upon priority among health care providers. However, this counseling is often done in a way that is perceived as coercive by patients – this was the experience of one of the young women quoted in the chapter on Voices of Lived Experience. She reported being shocked at the way in which the subject was introduced while she was still recovering from her delivery, when according to her, the last thing on her mind was becoming pregnant again or even having sex.

Long-acting reversible contraception (LARC) is safe and highly effective and is widely seen as the preferred mode for women of any age, including adolescents. It is also underutilized [18]. The utilization of this and other methods depends on their acceptance on the part of women at risk of repeat unwanted pregnancy. Accordingly, counseling about contraception should involve the presentation of sufficient information about available methods so that a shared decision-making process can occur within the context of patient preferences and medical history.

Advocacy

The Massachusetts Alliance on Teen Pregnancy is a model of an organization that advocated effectively for teen parents. The non-governmental organization was composed of teen parents (fathers as well as mothers).

For nearly 40 years, from 1979 to 2018, the Alliance advocated relentlessly on behalf of teen parents. Yearly demonstrations in front of the State House in Boston epitomized the politically savvy advocacy carried on by the Alliance. n 2011, the Alliance developed and implemented a new policy, *Expecting Success*, with specific recommendations to policymakers and educators on how to improve the educational attainment of teen parents to impact the trajectory of their lives and those of the young children they parent. Following the Expecting Success recommendations, Chelsea High School hired a part-time expectant and parenting student liaison for the 2011–2012 school year. As compared to the 2010–2011 school year, the *dropout rate among pregnant and parenting females decreased by 27%*. In addition, the liaison supported 89% of students who stayed at the high school for the 2011–2012 school year to graduate or achieve an on-time promotion.

> When asked what is the first step to [becoming] a successful teen mom they agreed that an education is what is most important.

The Alliance ended in 2018 with many aspects of its mission being institutionalized by the State, such as The Massachusetts Pregnant and Parenting Teen Initiative (MPPTI; https://www.mass.gov/the-massachusetts-pregnant-and-parenting-teen-initiative-mppti), which aims to increase life opportunities and enhance family stability among young families in the priority communities of Chelsea, Holyoke, Lawrence, New Bedford, and Springfield, or the Massachusetts Department of Public Health Sexual and Reproductive Health Program (https://www.mass.gov/sexual-and-reproductive-health-program-srhp), which aims to reduce unintended pregnancy and sexually transmitted infection rates by continually improving access to high quality education, outreach and clinical services through a statewide provider network and related special projects.

For many, the closing of the alliance in 2018 reflected the success of its efforts. In closing, the Alliance noted that Massachusetts had the third lowest teen birth rate in the nation (a goal consistent with teen pregnancy prevention) *but also* that more teen parents have stayed in school, received job training, and become self-supporting – achievements consistent with empowerment and respect, as opposed to stigma and shame.

Communities of Support

New models of service support for young mothers have arisen around the country. In Massachusetts, a particularly successful program over the last 20 years has been Connecting Young Moms (https://www.beverlyhospital.org/locations--services/health-services/obstetrics--maternity/young-moms-program), based in Beverly Hospital. Starting from a health education model (prenatal, then post-natal), this program has offered a host of clinical and social services and, especially important, through peer support groups, has created *communities of support,* groups of young mothers (and their children) who meet regularly, starting prenatally, for years – often finding a support community to replace what has been lost with family rejection.

Programs like Connecting Young Moms support young parents' having assets, i.e., factors in community, family, and self, that support growth and recovery. Newer programs also build on *assets,* seen as those protective elements in community, family, and in themselves, that help youth make informed choices and that support them, whichever choices they make. Peer supports are a major part of community supports.

Reducing Stigma Through Messaging

Within healthcare systems, educational institutions, and service organizations, inclusive policies may exist, but environments may still reflect stigmatizing messaging. Marketing materials such as posters, brochures, flyers, and banners should be reviewed for the following:

- Inclusive language that does not frame teen pregnancy or parenthood as a negative outcome.
- Sensitivity to racial and cultural stereotyping by ensuring photography reflects diversity and does not perpetuate stigma.
- Positive imagery of diverse family structures that do not uphold stereotypes of teen parent households, including positive imagery of single fathers, LGBTQ parents, and/or multi-generational homes.

Supporting the Education of Pregnant and Parenting Teens

There is universal agreement about the economic importance of education. For example, adults aged 18–64 in Massachusetts who attain their high school diploma or GED make $9249 more per year in mean annual earnings as compared to individuals who drop out [16].

Numerous studies have documented the lower SES, reduced earnings, and greater dependency on public support for many aspects of life, including health care (See, for example, the report of the Center for Labor Market Studies at Northeastern University and the Alternative Schools Network in Chicago, May [2]). This report warned, "The price of inaction will be increasing incarceration, welfare, high poverty rates among children, and healthcare costs for all USA taxpayers as dropouts and their families continue to fall through the cracks."

The high school dropout rate in the USA has been described over and over as a crisis; nearly one in four Americans and four in 10 minorities do not complete high school with their class [14]. While boys are more likely to drop out of school than girls, pregnancy or motherhood is one of the leading reasons why girls drop out, with 30% citing this as the reason. Only 40% of teen moms finish high school, and less than 2% of teen mothers (those who have a baby before age 18) finish college by age 30 (ibid.).

Policymakers have viewed preventing teen pregnancy as the major way of reducing dropout rates. While this is a worthwhile goal, it ignores the fact that for many teens, school is not very relevant to their daily lives and is not viewed as a pathway to a meaningful life. Indeed, motherhood presents a more attractive alternative for many of these young women, or "part of an alternative life-course strategy created in response to socioenvironmental constraints" ([1], p. 123). Efforts that focus exclusively on comprehensive sex education and reproductive health care will not change the appeal of school for teens who feel disconnected from their schools. These teens are not likely to return to a place that for them holds little hope of improving their lives. For many of those who do become pregnant and elect to carry their babies, school is often not a place they feel welcomed and supported, as we saw in the chapter on voices of lived experience. In that chapter, Natasha described how she was removed from honors classes and told that she should not apply to college after she became a parent.

A focus on improving schools' support for pregnant and parenting teens is a crucial component of keeping these young people in school. Given support and encouragement in school, a young mother can thrive, as we discussed in the chapter on interventions. Having a baby expands her horizons so that she thinks more about her future and that of her child, giving rise to a desire to be a good parent and provide opportunities for her child. Such a teen is likely to respond positively when the educational environment is encouraging and facilitating of her new role and her ability to succeed both as a parent and as a student. The following is one example of a policy to improve school support.

Boston Public Schools Expectant and Parenting Student Policy

- In 2014, the Boston Public Schools initiated a wide-ranging policy initiative, the Expectant and Parenting Student Policy (https://www.bostonpublicschools.org/domain/2610), which emphasizes support and respect for students who become parents (2014). In developing the policy, with support from the Mass Alliance for Teen Pregnancy, the district collaborated with expectant and parenting students, medical professionals, and service organization providers to improve the policy and include the following: Inclusive language: Young parents deserve to be recognized and respected for their roles as parents regardless of their gender identity. In the policy, gender-inclusive terms like "parents and co-parents of all genders" were used rather than only mothers and fathers.
- Maintain confidentiality: Expectant and parenting students' autonomy is upheld by allowing them to choose how and when to inform parents, relatives, caregivers, as well as seek services and support. School staff must follow all applicable laws on student confidentiality. Expectant and parenting students may not be pressured, forced or coerced to tell their parents or any other person of their expectant or parenting status.
- Ensure a safe, supportive learning environment: Expectant and parenting students are explicitly protected from being excluded from any school, program, class, or activity on the basis of their expectant and/or parenting status. Expectant and parenting students have the right to attend school in an environment free of discrimination, judgment, and harassment.
- Promote academic success: The choice to enroll in an alternative school or program must be completely voluntary and school staff are expected to maintain high expectations for student success. A student cannot be pressured or coerced to leave their current educational environment for another. In addition, school-based student support staff should collaborate with the student to develop an academic plan within their own defined goals.
- Implement sensible attendance policies: Absences related to pregnancy are considered excused absences for expectant students. In the policy, student parents are entitled to a fair and reasonable parental leave after the birth of a child and may take excused absences when their child is sick or has a medical appointment during school hours. Schools are encouraged to work with expectant and parenting students to determine a school schedule that promotes regular and on-time attendance without fear of penalization.

- Use liaisons to share information: Schools with any grades 6–12 should identify a school liaison for expectant and parenting students to help funnel resources and share information about their rights. Liaisons can be responsible for informing the school community about the policy too.
- If a district already has an Expectant and Parenting Student Policy, it is possible it may be outdated or lack inclusive language or sufficient detail about the rights and responsibilities of schools and students. Work with local parenting students, community members, and service providers to update and implement a new policy.
- If there is no expectant and parenting student policy in place, develop one with parenting students, community members, and local service providers to ensure young parents receive equitable access to resources to ensure they are empowered to stay in school and graduate.

Summary

Historically, negative stereotypes about teen parents, often influenced by racist beliefs, have guided public policy initiatives related to teen pregnancy, with a result that pregnant and parenting teens have been stigmatized and treated in a punitive manner rather than given the support that would enable them and their children to thrive. Changing attitudes is not easy, as the current efforts to combat racism have shown. It requires empathy and listening to those who have been stigmatized. Public policy has tended to focus much more on prevention, whether improving access to contraception and abortion or promoting abstinence than on providing support for young parents. These negative policies have persisted despite numerous examples of effective programs that do help these young people succeed both as parents and as developing individuals. And, in many cases, the voices of the young people themselves about what they need and want have not been heard. This is starting to change, part of a paradigm of change in the fields of medicine and social services, in which recipients of services are treated as collaborative partners with service providers rather than passive beneficiaries. Ideally efforts to prevent pregnancy should be balanced with interventions *after* pregnancy. Policies that empower and support young parents are not meant to and do not endorse or encourage teen pregnancy. They are not designed to replace initiatives to prevent pregnancy, but rather to complement them. These new policies seek to put the decision about becoming parents in the hands of the young people themselves, while supporting the *assets* that help them make good choices for themselves and for the next generation. They are the result of listening to the voices of lived experience.

References

1. Burton LM (Teenage childbearing as an alternative life-course strategy in multigeneration black families. Hum Nat. 1990;1(2):123–43. https://doi.org/10.1007/BF02692149.

2. Center for Labor Market Studies at Northeastern University and the Alternative Schools Network in Chicago. Left behind in America: the Nation's dropout crisis. Boston, MA: Author; 2009, May.
3. Cook S, Cameron S. Social issues of teenage pregnancy. Obstet Gynaecol Reprod Med. 2015;25:243–8. https://doi.org/10.1016/j.ogrm.2015.06.001.
4. Denno DM, Hoopes AJ, Chandra-Mouli V. Effective strategies to provide adolescent sexual and reproductive health services and to increase demand and community support. J Adolesc Health. 2015;56(1):S22–41. https://doi.org/10.1016/j.jadohealth.2014.09.012.
5. Dyck JJ, Hussey LS. The end of welfare as we know it? Public Opin Q. 2008;72(4):589–618. https://doi.org/10.1093/poq/nfn053.
6. Edin K, Shaefer L. 20 years since welfare 'reform'. The Atlantic; 2016, 22 August 2016.
7. Fleming N, O'Driscoll T, Becker G, Spitzer RF. Adolescent pregnancy guidelines. J Obstet Gynaecol Can. 2015;37(8):740–56. https://www.bostonpublicschools.org/domain/2610. https://doi.org/10.1016/S1701-2163(15)30180-8.
8. Harper G. Child and adolescent mental health policy. In: Rey J, editor. IACAPAP e-Textbook on child and adolescent mental health. International Association for Child and Adolescent Psychiatry and Allied Professions; 2012. https://iacapap.org.
9. Institute of Medicine Committee on Quality of Health Care in America. Crossing the quality chasm: a new health system for the 21st century. Washington, DC: National Academy Press; 2001.
10. Kuhn T. The structure of scientific revolutions. 2nd ed. Chicago: University of Chicago Press; 1970.
11. Mason-Jones AJ, Sinclair D, Mathews C, Kagee A, Hillman A, Lombard C. School-based interventions for preventing HIV, sexually transmitted infections, and pregnancy in adolescents. Cochrane Database Syst Rev. 2016;11(11):CD006417. https://doi.org/10.1002/14651858.CD006417.pub3.
12. National Association of State Legislators. State policies on sex education in schools. 2020. https://www.ncsl.org/research/health/state-policies-on-sex-education-in-schools.aspx.
13. Stanger-Hall KF, Hall DW. Abstinence-only education and teen pregnancy rates: Why we need comprehensive sex education in the U.S. PloS One. 2011;6(10):e24658. https://doi.org/10.1371/journal.pone.0024658.
14. Shuger L. Teen Pregnancy and High School Dropout: What Communities Can Do to Address These Issues. 2012; Washington, DC: The National Campaign to Prevent Teen and Unplanned Pregnancy and America's Promise Alliance. https://powertodecide.org/sites/default/files/resources/primary-download/teen-pregnancy-and-high-school-dropout.pdf.
15. Stephan P. Research efficiency: perverse incentives. Nature. 2012;484(7392):29–31. https://doi-org.ezp-prod1.hul.harvard.edu/10.1038/484029a
16. Sum A, Khatiwada I, McLaughlin J, Tobar P. An assessment of the labor market, income, health, social, civic and fiscal consequences of dropping out of high school: findings for Massachusetts adults in the 21st century. Boston, Massachusetts: Northeastern University; 2007. http://hdl.handle.net/2047/d10015280
17. Talbot M. Red sex, blue sex: Why do so many evangelical teenagers become pregnant? New Yorker. 2008; https://www.newyorker.com/magazine/2008/11/03/red-sex-blue-sex.
18. Wu JP, Moniz MH, Ursu AN. Long-acting reversible contraception – highly efficacious, safe, and underutilized. JAMA. 2018;320(4):397–8. https://doi.org/10.1001/jama.2018.8877.
19. Yang Z, Gaydos LM. Reasons for and challenges of recent increases in teen birth rates: a study of family planning service policies and demographic changes at the state level. J Adolesc Health. 2010;46(6):517–24.

Conclusions

11

Jean-Victor P. Wittenberg

Introduction

This book's focus and content were influenced by many individuals over a long period of time. The history of our group includes a monograph *titled Crises of Adolescence*, now over 35 years old [3]. Our initial goal was to provide an update to the 1986 monograph, with the aim of advocating for the health and development of young mothers, fathers, and their babies. As we worked to understand teen pregnancy in a contemporary context, we became more and more aware of the role that stigma plays in teen pregnancy—that is, its destructive effects on teen parents and their children. We strove to identify the processes through which stigma works in our communities, our social agencies, our professional offices, our research, our policies, practices, and even in our laws. This led us to focus this time on stigma and the dynamics of its power in harming adolescents who were more likely to become pregnant because of stigma, those who do become pregnant, and their babies. Reading it now, we can see where stigma—accepted beliefs and practices of the Committee at that time—appears in our 1986 monograph. In time, we may find that we too have stigmatizing beliefs that need to change; we will welcome such changes.

Our work has taken on a degree of urgency in the context of the pandemic. Prior to the pandemic we often did not openly recognize and acknowledge the appalling impact of our own biases on our neighbors. These biases—stigma—are to be found in individual encounters and cultural beliefs, in traditional practices and documented policies. The pandemic, the ACE studies, and stress research have made it clear that being part of a marginalized population, whether defined by skin color, by poverty, by disability, by gender identity, etc., makes one more likely to live a more

J.-V. P. Wittenberg (✉)
University of Toronto, Toronto, ON, Canada

Hospital for Sick Children, Toronto, ON, Canada
e-mail: jean.wittenberg@sickkids.ca

J.-V. P. Wittenberg et al. (eds.), *Adolescent Pregnancy and Parenting*,
https://doi.org/10.1007/978-3-031-42502-8_11

stressed life, to live a shorter life, to be vulnerable to severe challenges to health and development from infancy to the end of life. Marginalized populations suffer these consequences as a direct result of stigma; the consequences have been aggravated by the pandemic but were imposed prior to the pandemic and independent of it. Teen parents and their children are a marginalized population.

Population studies have shown us the phenomenon of stigma against adolescent mothers is world-wide and that teen birth rates are an important metric of adolescent health globally (UNESCO). Although some populations accept and nurture the children, most are very critical of their adolescent mothers. In past years we have seen a sustained and significant global decrease in rates of teen pregnancy and yet teen pregnancy continues to account for more than 10% of global births. The vast majority occur in low- or middle-income nations but curiously, among wealthy nations, the USA has the highest rate of teen mothers. [6]. Teen pregnancy and adolescent parents pose issues for western communities as much as anywhere else in the world; attitudes to teen parenthood vary across national borders and within national states and provinces [9].

Stigma is strongly associated with adverse health outcomes [4]. Stigma is an attribute of human nature that has served many functions, at times promoting social cohesion, but also associated with perpetuating power gradients. It supports traditions, policies, and practices held by a more powerful social group targeting a weaker group; protecting the advantages of the more privileged group and keeping disadvantaged individuals and groups lower on the social gradient. We know that being low on the social gradient is associated with multiple undesirable consequences—clearly for individuals, and for communities. It costs us more, as individuals and as communities, to live with stigma than to recognize it.

Stigmatizing beliefs are built on foundations of misinformation and disinformation. They are demonstrably untrue. When social disadvantage is controlled for, populations do not differ in capacity and achievement. Stigmatizing beliefs are often unconscious but can also be overt and have been dramatically illuminated by Black Lives Matter. Stigma mistakenly defines others as different, inferior, even threatening. Others are seen as alien—the enemy.

Our review of the literature and our discussions with adolescent parents (reviewed in our Chap. 2) make it clear that these are individuals who, for multiple intersecting and compounding reasons, have become parents in adolescence. They are more likely to have been poor, racialized, have disabilities, been exposed to violence, maltreatment, child welfare, family mental health disorders, had fewer opportunities that promote health, education, etc. The religious and political environments of communities also affect rates. Policies, such as those that affect sex education and access to contraception and abortion, are crucial determinants of teen birth rates. It has been very clearly demonstrated that the most effective way to decrease rates of teen pregnancy is by providing education, access to birth control, and other supportive social and educational measures. Nonetheless, stigmatizing beliefs lead us to blame them for what teens do all over the world; they have sex. It is clearly a normal behavior for adolescents. Can we not ask how we can help them to health and safety rather than condemn them for what we ourselves and all our ancestors have been doing for all time?

Hearing the Voices of Adolescent Parents

Research and our own experiences of working with adolescent parents have shown us that many adolescent parents have capacity and promise. Many succeed; they have jobs, raise children, etc. All too often, to succeed, they have had to overcome challenges imposed by stigmatizing social attitudes. The teens ask: How are they to continue getting an education? How are they to hold a job? How are they to maintain familial and peer relationships? How are they to maintain a sense of personal worth and goals? The teens themselves and the research literature tell us that many fail to meet standards their advantaged age cohort meet, but that often they exceed the standards of their equally disadvantaged peers. We ask how many more might succeed were it not for the stresses that stigma has imposed?

Perhaps the most important lesson for all of us has been to hear the voices of teen parents. Informed understanding depends on evidence. If we do not heed those voices, we exclude indispensable data. Teen parents tell us repeatedly, when we are open to asking open-ended questions and hearing their answers, that stigma affects all aspects of their lives. Studies have documented that stigma affects not only the teens themselves, but also their children and even the children's grandparents. Stigma has robbed them of resources and subjected them to stressful encounters on the street, in public transit, in supermarkets, shops and malls, in schools, and in daycares. It leads to stress in the offices of health care service providers. Stigma leaves them without resources, with few choices and limited opportunities.

Not all teen pregnancies are unplanned and those that are planned involve a calculus that considers social and cultural conditions resulting in the decision to have a child. For these teens, the decision is an "alternative life-course strategy" [1]. Studies show us that a significant number, when they become pregnant, make changes that make them more productive members of our communities [8]. They change their housing, continue their education, develop careers, and become independent wage earners based on a new sense of perspective in life, a commitment to self-improvement and devotion to the well-being of their children. The baby gives them meaning and direction in life.

Stigma, however, creates negative self-representations. Negative attitudes are attributed to them by their families, teachers, others, even their peers. They cope by submitting/complying ("I accept that I am bad") or by opposing them. That healthy opposition can then be interpreted as to "prove" negative social attitudes to them [4]. These negative self-representations appear in the attitudes of their peers to pregnant or mothering adolescents [5]. Many interventions are peer driven; there is a risk that stigma compromises the effectiveness of those supports.

Developmental Issues: Adolescent Mothers and Fathers

Adolescence and infancy/early childhood are pivotal periods for development. The infant's experiences before the age of 2 years predict lifespan outcomes. Brain function, emotional, cognitive, and behavioral regulation are in *status nascendi.* The same is true for the adolescent. The adolescent brain is just getting to a state in which it can support a stable sense of identity [2, 7]. The development of critical brain pathways and skill acquisition establish trajectories for the lifespan for both the infant and the adolescent. Both infant and adolescent are qualitatively different as they emerge into childhood and adulthood.

Teen pregnancy and parenthood challenge two separate but interacting lines of development: identity formation (vs. role confusion; Erikson) and parenting, perhaps more for teen mothers but also for teen fathers. For some teens, the two lines of development create conflict but for some becoming pregnant provides them with meaning and direction that supports identity.

Erikson saw life stages as involving a conflict between individual needs and societal demands. We would argue that each stage also depends on the availability of social supports. As Erikson saw it, each developmental phase has its own crisis; successful resolution of the crisis results in new strengths and capacities, however, developmental transitions can result in emotional growth or can be disorganizing. Optimal development requires age-appropriate relationships and social support leading to the development of life skills and capacities. Social supports are particularly important for adolescents and thus stigma, which attacks one's social self, is more likely to have adverse effects at this age. At younger ages we depend more on our parents for self-esteem. In adulthood, if we have established a sense of identity, we can sustain our own self-esteem more effectively.

Identity formation and parenting depend on the development of some similar capacities. We have considered two: executive function (EF) and reflective function (RF). EF, solving problems using cognitive skills including the capacity to tolerate delay, restrain impulses, consider consequences, etc., is acquired over the course of development and can be overwhelmed by stress or by desire. The surge in the development of cognitive capacity in adolescence provides an improved foundation for EF but the ability to regulate desire and impulsiveness develops more slowly. The increased incidence of risk-taking in adolescence perfectly demonstrates the vulnerability of executive function at that age; not only does that vulnerability make them more likely, for example, to engage in unprotected sex but it also makes them prone to making impulsive decisions in the face of stress imposed from others including the baby. For many teens, disadvantage includes strife in the family of origin, increased likelihood of mental health problems, and other characteristics that interfere with the optimal development of EF and of emotional regulation. Other family members are likely to feel the impact of stigmatizing beliefs in their day-to-day encounters as well although most is more likely attributable to factors other than the teen pregnancy. That stress is part of the toxic soup many of these families live in, stress that impacts them as well as the teen parent and the baby.

With parenthood come social expectations to manage tasks beyond those demanded of most adolescents: e.g., housing, arranging financial support or getting a job, planning a budget, working with daycare and healthcare professionals for the baby, etc. The teens need support and guidance as they come to make decisions, respect to decide their own futures and support to carry out their plans. Effective interventions require individualized and comprehensive approaches as well as rigorous evaluation to assess usefulness to both mothers and children.

Many can be expected to encounter child welfare agencies. Child welfare intrusion into the life of a parent is a hugely threatening event that demands high degrees of problem-solving on the part of the parents. Some agencies are re-conceptualizing their roles—working to empower teen parents, as well as other parents they work with such as First Nations parents in Canada, Black parents across North America. They work to understand the circumstances that brought these families to child welfare attention and seek out the strengths and promise in the parents. This is another example of correcting previously stigmatizing beliefs.

RF, the capacity to consider one's own mind as well as the mind of the other in interactions, is also very much in development through adolescence. Optimal parenting demands parental awareness of the infant's and child's mind. The development of RF is less well studied in adolescence, but it is clear that RF depends on the regulation that EF provides. Intense urges and feelings, high levels of stress and impulsiveness interfere with RF.

The perspective of teen fathers is rarely sought in determining policy or when we make clinical decisions. Clinical appointments for mothers and babies rarely permit, let alone invite, fathers' participation. They are too often seen as if all these fathers were the same—all seeking impulsive sexual gratification and wanting nothing to do with the responsibility of fatherhood. They are described as absent and uninterested in the mothers or babies. However, there is much variability among teen fathers. We know that fathers can be a strength in the teen family system but our excluding them can compromise their contribution and even further, can be psychologically harmful to the fathers who do wish to be involved. When fathers do remain involved, better outcomes for the children are more likely. Fathers can provide an important source of support and self-esteem for mothers. They can be present when all other peers have disappeared.

Family support for teen parents is a two-edged sword; it can be very supportive and protective, but it can also interfere and condemn the teens. Given the degree of stress that many families experience, stress that is often aggravated by the birth of a new baby, relationships can be fraught with difficulty and conflict. The relationships can support development of maternal/paternal skills and confidence in the parents, or it can rob them of confidence. Grandparents may undermine their own children through taking over the care of the new baby themselves, rather than understanding and expressing trust in the teen parent(s) and supporting their growth and development. This is a difficult situation in which the teens' stage of development, anxiety about being a parent and willingness to give up that responsibility may conspire with grandparents taking over. Both the teen parent and the baby need support for optimal physical, cognitive, and relational development.

Mental Health Conditions and Substance Use

The psychosocial stressors many teen parents face because of poverty, marginalization, and stigma—compounded by the stresses of pregnancy and parenthood—place them at risk for a variety of emotional and psychological problems. Many of them are at high risk for problems that will permanently impact their quality of life as well as their children's lives.

Mental health conditions constitute both pre-existing conditions, which are risk factors for teen pregnancy as well as consequences of it. These conditions also greatly impact the children born to affected parents. Young parents are particularly at risk for both prenatal and perinatal depression, a common disorder that has many negative effects on both parents and children. Effective treatments are available, but conditions must be identified first. Tools for routine screening for depression, anxiety, and substance use disorders in primary care and obstetrical settings are available and professional and governmental organizations have advocated for their use.

Substance use deserves particular emphasis, both because of its potential to have devastating effects on infants and children, but also because pregnancy and the perinatal period are ideal times to intervene. Like pre-existing mental health conditions, substance use is a risk factor for unplanned pregnancy. How careful are we to identify mental health and substance use problems as health issues rather than as moral failures?

Infant Development and Outcomes

As a group, offspring of adolescent mothers fare more poorly in terms of physical and mental health, development, education, vocation, relationships, etc. than the children of older mothers, for many reasons. These disadvantages begin in pregnancy and perhaps even earlier, before conception. Once again, we emphasize that there are no simple answers as to causation. All outcomes are determined by many influences, however, as we learn more, it becomes apparent that excessive maternal stress plays a part, and that stigma contributes to this stress. There is good evidence of stress changing the placental interface leading to more highly stressed newborns, newborns with lower birth weights and lower APGAR scores. When parents are stressed, they are more likely to emit more distressing signals that are perceived and responded to by infants and children. Stigma increases those interactions between parents and children; those interactions are associated with higher levels of psychopathology in infants and children into their adult years. It is clear from the ACE studies, that excessive, prolonged experiences of stress in infancy and childhood are associated with severe lifespan health consequences.

Poverty and lack of social supports characterize very large numbers of teen-parent-led families. These cause stress to parents and directly to infants and children. Teen mothers report feeling targeted by stigmatizing, stress-inducing social attitudes that also influence provision of care by health care service professionals. Teen mothers are more likely to avoid making or attending medical appointments.

Empowering Pregnant and Parenting Adolescents

It is crucial that service providers examine their own beliefs and attitudes about teen parents. Although it is very common for healthcare and social service providers to have negative expectations about them, most teen parents have a desire to do well for their children's sake and supporting them in this goal should be the essence of interventions. Regarding both prevention and intervention, empowerment is important. What this means is emphasizing agency, through identification and support of strengths rather than focusing on deficits. Training for personnel in schools, clinics and social welfare agencies can help to increase awareness of stigmatizing attitudes and practices among teachers, health care providers, and aid workers.

Pregnancy and parenting in adolescence are associated with higher risk for adverse outcomes, but adverse outcomes are not inevitable. As we saw in earlier chapters, some young parents do better than their peers from similar circumstances who do not have children. As we described in the chapter on interventions, there are several evidence-based resources and programs that can help empower adolescents to better care for themselves and their children and improve outcomes. The most efficacious of these programs empower young parents to improve their lives and the lives of their children. These programs include school-based programs, home visiting programs, community outreach, embedded services in the medical home, and co-parenting groups. These programs can help to decrease the stigma of adolescent pregnancy, reinforce help-seeking behaviors, encourage parents to stay in school, and improve parental competency. Advocacy for funding of these programs and for medically accurate sexual education and use of contraception should be a priority.

Providers in programs for teens and their babies should look at individual risk factors and help parents decide their goals and access appropriate resources. Both the individuals and their social contexts are important in assessment—both need to be addressed in interventions. There is a great deal of heterogeneity among young parents and programs need to be culturally sensitive and tailored to specific communities. "One size fits all" is not a good approach. Seeking autonomy is a healthy characteristic of adolescence that needs to be fostered. Seeking, understanding, and responding to input from the teens involved is indispensable in both program planning and design and in individual interventions.

Policy

Public policy is meant to express and implement the values of the community or organization but is developed at a point in time. Understanding, perspective, and values change over time and thus policies need repeated re-evaluation and adaptation. It is instructive to examine policies that are in place and to assess their impact on well-researched evidence. Clearly many present-day policies do not support and empower young parents in their roles as parents and as emerging adults; rather they express stigmatizing views and impose stress on teen parents and as a result on their babies and children. Unfortunately, all too often polices are created without consultation with the individuals impacted by the practices those policies support. Those policies and practices lead to paradoxical outcomes as has been the case leading to more school dropouts, more teen pregnancies, more child poverty as outlined in our chapter on Policy. The opposite can also be true, such as was the case with the Massachusetts Alliance on Teen Pregnancy, where information was taken from pregnant and mothering teens to effect policy. Policy has life-changing power affecting millions, with the potential to improve health and lives or to blight them and impose costs and unwanted consequences on all of us.

Stigma distorts our perceptions, our research, our policies, and our practices. Careful, scientifically rigorous, evaluation of policies and practices are indispensable to good health delivery. The science must address the heterogeneity of the populations involved and consider various life-trajectory choices; there is more than one way to live a life. Research, policy, and practice must include the voices of those most closely involved from inception through design and implementation. Salient outcomes in this population begin with the questions they themselves ask and the outcomes that concern them. We must also include assessment of health and development for teen parents and their children, short-term and most critically, long-term costs to communities associated with different policies and practices.

We must each ask ourselves how we perceive our patients and clients. We must recall that we as service providers are in positions of power. Stigma, when associated with power, causes harm. Beyond our own individual efforts, we must also examine the power gradients in healthcare, social service delivery, education, and policy. Stigma does not change without changes in those power gradients. Stigma causes as much or more ill health as any virus or bacterium, any of the public health risks and occupational hazards we encounter. Our own commitment to the practice of good healthcare means that we have a responsibility to address the health impact of stigma.

References

1. Burton LM. Teenage childbearing as an alternative life-course strategy in multigeneration black families. Human Nature 1. 1990;123–43. https://doi.org/10.1007/BF02692149.
2. Erikson EH. Identity, youth and crisis. New York, NY: W. W. Norton & Company, Inc; 1968.
3. Group for the Advancement of Psychiatry. Crises of adolescence. Teenage pregnancy: impact on adolescent development. New York: Brunner/Mazel; 1986.
4. Hatzenbuehler ML, Phelan JC, Link BG. Stigma as a fundamental cause of population health inequalities. Am J Public Health. 2013;103(5):813–21. https://doi.org/10.2105/AJPH.2012.301069. Epub 2013 Mar 14. PMID: 23488505; PMCID: PMC3682466.
5. Jones C, Whitfield C, Seymour J, Hayter M. 'Other girls': a qualitative exploration of teenage mothers' views on teen pregnancy in contemporaries. Sex C. 2019;23(3):760–73.
6. Olszewski L, Diaz A. Adolescent parenting: global perspective, local action. Annal Glob Health. 2019;85(1):62. https://doi.org/10.5334/aogh.2477.
7. Romeo RD. The teenage brain: the stress response and the adolescent brain. Curr Dir Psychol Sci. 2013;22(2):140–5. https://doi-org.ezp-prod1.hul.harvard.edu/10.1177/0963721413475445

8. SmithBattle L. Reframing the risks and losses of teen mothering. MCN Am J Matern Child Nurs. 2009;34(2):122–8. https://doi.org/10.1097/01.NMC.0000347307.93079.7d. PMID: 19262267.
9. Talbot M. Red sex, blue sex: why do so many evangelical teenagers become pregnant? New Yorker, October 27 2008. https://www.newyorker.com/magazine/2008/11/03/red-sex-blue-sex

Index

J. P. -V. Wittenberg et al. (eds.), *Adolescent Pregnancy and Parenting*,
https://doi.org/10.1007/978-3-031-42502-8

MIX
Papier aus verantwortungsvollen Quellen
Paper from responsible sources
FSC® C105338

If you have any concerns about our products,
you can contact us on
ProductSafety@springernature.com

In case Publisher is established outside the EU,
the EU authorized representative is:
Springer Nature Customer Service Center GmbH
Europaplatz 3, 69115 Heidelberg, Germany

Printed by Libri Plureos GmbH
in Hamburg, Germany